I Am Your Mirror

Mirror Neurons and Empathy

Matteo Rizzato and Davide Donelli

Introduction by Prof. Giacomo Rizzolatti

I Am Your Mirror

Mirror Neurons and Empathy

Translation: Stefano Cozzi
Art cover: Amritagraphic

blossomingbooks

First published 2014 by
Blossoming Books:
www.blossomingbooks.com

Blossoming Books is a trademark of Edizioni Amrita srl

Edizioni Amrita srl
Via San Quintino, 36
10121 Torino - Italy
www.amrita-edizioni.com

Printed in United States of America

TO OUR READERS

The books that we publish represent our contribution to an emerging world that is based upon a spirit of cooperation rather than competitiveness, as well as upon the progressive establishment of the human spirit instead of casting doubts on its true value, coupled with the certainty that all individuals are interconnected. Our goal is to reach out and touch as many lives as possible by conveying to them a message of hope for a better world.

Behind each of our books lie many hours of enthusiastic work, great care and thorough investigation, commencing with the choice of which titles to publish, determined by our reading committee, through a meticulously accurate translation process, and often long and absorbing investigations by the editorial team.

We would like our readers to be aware of all this, so that they can really taste not only the contents of this book, but also all the love and dedication involved in bringing it to fruition.

The publishers

Praise for

I Am Your Mirror
Mirror Neurons and Empathy

"This work is a must read for anyone involved in the mediation or crisis intervention field; or for that matter, anyone who must interact with people on a daily basis. People are inclined to manage psychological distress by believing in the credibility of those whom they must depend upon to get them through their misfortune. Rizzato and Donelli have provided a blueprint for motivating human behavior by providing awareness of our own telegraphed mannerisms and gestures, and have brought basic active listening skills into the third dimension. By mirroring positive and empathic emotions in difficult encounters, people will almost always respond with promising outcomes."

~ *Lieutenant Jack J. Cambria*
Commanding Officer, NYPD Hostage Negotiation Team

"Science, psychology, and sociology merge to explain the theory of the biology of empathy...People often mirror one another's emotions...If people are more aware of their influence, they could become more positive, unite humankind, and build a brighter world..."

~ *ForeWord Reviews*

"This book is a reminder to everyone who works in healthcare of how their behavior affects everyone they meet. Compassionate healthcare providers can improve the outlook of patients, caregivers and family members who are often burdened with negative emotions."

~ *Richard Cheu*
Author of Living Well with Chronic Illness
Neurophysiologist – Hospital Chaplain

"In *I Am Your Mirror*, Rizzato and Donelli take a potentially complex topic and make it extremely accessible to any reader. The book is wonderfully engaging as it both educates its readers about the science of mirror neurons, as well as offers practical advice for individuals to improve the quality of their daily interactions."

~ *Jocelyn Elise Crowley, Ph.D.*
Professor of Public Policy, Rutgers, The State University of New Jersey
Author of Mothers Unite!, The Politics of Child Support in America, *&* Defiant Dads

"This is a gem of a book because it packs the treasures of new science in a brief format...Reaching across levels from tiny neurons to world peace, *I Am Your Mirror* is destined to become a valuable addition to many educational formats..."

~ *Johanna Wolfson, Ph.D.*
California Board of Psychology Licensed Psychologist
Albert Einstein School of Medicine of Yeshiva University Graduate

Praise for *I Am Your Mirror* VII
Foreword.................... 1
Authors' introduction.................... 5

Chap. 1 - What are mirror neurons? 9
Preamble 9
A few concepts 10
The way we function 18
Function, not form 22
Visual motor neurons 25
Objects? No, hypotheses! 26
Action vocabulary 28
Spatial representation 31
Mirror neurons 33
The function of mirror neurons 37
Intention 39
What are you doing? 43
I cannot see? In that case I will listen! 46
Understanding 47
Vocabulary differences 48
The role of emotions 50
Chap. 2 - A daily discovery 57
Let's talk about us 57
What kind of face are you pulling? 59

We have always imitated each other 60
We watch, and then we try 63
Social responsibility 67
Chap. 3 - Observation: an instrument for action 73
We improve through observation 73
Observing and acting 76
Innate imitation 79
Acting appropriately 82
Act within groups 85
Hello? 87
Chap. 4 - Congruence and emotions 91
Imitating sincerity 91
Congruence 92
Nuances and strategies 95
The war of the neurons 99

Conclusion 103
About the authors 109
Acknowledgements 111
Bibliography 113
More... 113

FOREWORD

This book is an excellent choice for those wanting a simple, straightforward introduction to mirror neurons and their functions. Its origin goes back a couple of years to when Davide Donelli, a medical student at the University of Parma, Italy, asked to come and see me for a chat. I thought that he might ask me for an explanation of some of the topics contained in my human physiology course, but it turned out that his request was totally different. Donelli wanted my opinion in relation to an initiative that he intended to pursue in conjunction with Dr. Matteo Rizzato, a professional coach who operates in Italy's Friuli region. Their idea was to write a book that would bring "the mirror neuron mechanism and its implications in everyday life to the level of understanding of ordinary people". I must confess that I was somewhat puzzled: I knew that Rizzato had taken an interest in mirror neurons, in that he had actually written a reply–and in so doing, had shown a high degree of expertise–to an article published by the *Gazzettino* newspaper, in which a Professor of Engineering from Udine had scribbled a lot of nonsense about mirror neurons. Nonetheless, although the level of knowledge of these two authors was complementary and could therefore set the book on an interesting course, I remained sceptical, as neither of them was a neuroscientist. Nevertheless, my reply to them was: "Give it a go".

Around a year had gone by when the two authors asked for an appointment and came to give me their finished manuscript. I read a few sections at random and found that its style was pleasant and its presentation accurate; I was also really struck by its illustrations, which were beautifully done, amusing and scientifically accurate. Sometimes a picture can explain a concept better than a thousand words. I congratulated the two authors, but reserved the right to read the entire book in order to provide them with a more in-depth opinion and to remove any possible errors and inaccuracies that a non-professional might have possibly overlooked.

Due to lack of time on my part, it was a while before I could return the book to its authors, who had been patiently waiting–and now that the (few) errors and inaccuracies have been corrected, the reader can have confidence in the information contained herein, even though it was not written by a team of specialists, but rather by two enthusiasts in the field.

As the authors themselves have stated, the book consists essentially of two parts: the first section is based upon the book *Mirrors in the Brain*[1], which Corrado Sinigaglia and myself co-wrote a few years ago. This section provides some basic information on mirror neurons and their characteristics, in addition to presenting some simple neurophysiological notions required for understanding the way mirror neurons operate. The second section deals with the application of this knowledge to everyday life, and this is the most original part of this

1 G. Rizzolatti, C. Sinigaglia, *Mirrors in the Brain. How Our Minds Share Actions and Emotions*, Oxford University Press, 2007.

book, where the reader will find some interesting advice on how to behave appropriately in certain circumstances, taking into account the responses of others' mirror neurons. I cannot possibly know whether after reading this book its readers will behave better towards others, but at least they will be able to understand why some of their reactions may end up producing different results from those intended.

Should readers develop an interest in this subject matter, they can extend their knowledge by consulting some books that contain more detailed descriptions of the experiments and present a deeper analysis of the theoretical aspects that have brought us to the conclusions described here. This book, however, represents an excellent starting point. I recommend it.

Giacomo Rizzolatti

AUTHORS' INTRODUCTION

Knowing each other as we do, we have discovered that we have many things in common, and one of these in particular has driven us to write this book, namely the discovery of mirror neurons. To be honest, this event has had a deep influence on our lives, both personally and professionally. Our intent was to create a book that was easy to read and geared towards those who wished to understand as clearly as possible the potential represented by the discovery of these so-called mirrors, while examining them in the course of their daily activities.

Mirror neurons are cells in our brain that enable us to perform an extremely important task: *to trace back all that we perceive and all that we are capable of doing to a common format*. What does this mean? In practical terms, this means that when we see another person carry out a certain action, the mirror neurons inside us become activated, and they make us 'live' the observed action, just as if we were carrying it out ourselves.

This explains why, whenever we observe someone yawning, we automatically imitate that person. We can reproduce the action because, at the moment that we see it, that very same gesture is present within us, as if it were us who were doing it, with just one difference: it is present inside us only at the level of potential. It is actually our will that subsequently transforms that potential gesture into an actual one. Even so, whether we like it or not, when we observe others, mirror neurons are preparing us to experience from within the very thing that we are observing.

Clearly the debate has acquired a much wider scope after the revelation that mirror neurons are also applicable to *emotion*: there is in us a 'Mirror System' capable of associating the image of people we are observing with the emotions that they are experiencing, thus making us live, even if only partially perhaps, the same precise sensations of those we are observing, and this is especially the case for *negative* emotions.

This is why, when we find ourselves in the presence of other people, our space then becomes a *shared space* in which, thanks to this extraordinary mechanism in our brain, inevitably *our actions and emotions are immediately recognised and understood by others.* This profoundly unites us, because it is scientific confirmation that *we cannot help experiencing what is experienced by whoever is around us.* And vice versa.

The discovery of both mirror neurons and the Mirror System is the result of the research carried out over the last thirty years by a group of distinguished Italian scientists, namely Fogassi, Fadiga, Gallese and Di Pellegrino, co-ordinated by Professor Giacomo Rizzolatti. The members of this amazing team have been able–owing to their ability to go beyond the traditional patterns of neurophysiological research–to gain access to this extraordinary mechanism in our brain, the discovery of which is now deeply affecting not only the scientific environment, but also the lives of ordinary people and the way they see themselves within the context of their surrounding world. Have you ever noticed those photographs displayed on desks in the workplace? And have you ever wondered why those specific ones have been chosen? And what about those that some of us carry in our wallets, or use as screensavers on our computers or mobile phones?

These are just some of the questions that this book tries to find answers to and correlations, starting from an approach supplied by scientific studies and connecting them to everyday actions.

We have chosen to make use of real and tangible examples that can demonstrate the incredible interactions that exist between mirror neurons and individual's actions on a practical level. The sheer level of conditioning that these connections exert over human behaviour is astonishing.

The goal of this book is essentially to provide everyone with a direct and easy to use set of tools with which to begin immediately to observe, recognise and manage this discovery's basic levels of functionality within the framework of interpersonal relationships. This is done by making use of everything that we are able to observe in our daily practice, that is to say in all the small actions that we all perform.

After reading many texts with the scientific details of these studies, we became convinced that such an extraordinary discovery could not be exclusively confined to the understanding of a few selected individuals through a bibliography that was heavily centred on the scientific and biological dynamics of this subject. In our opinion (which we like to regard as that of two incurable pioneers and researchers in the field of those discoveries that increase human knowledge) it was important to add one more voice, a different kind of interpretation from what may otherwise emerge from such a significant step forward in the field of neuroscience. We believe it is *crucial* that the awareness that originates from this discovery be shared among all, in that it helps us understand an important part of how we function and can consequently result in an appreciable improvement in our relationships with others, and above all with ourselves.

This book is divided into two parts, the first of which deals with the subject of mirror neurons by presenting a sort of 'basic manual' on the matter; while the second part shares what has been learned from the direct experience of applying these research studies to the world of training, education and consultancy. The first part provides some basic scientific notions, and then goes on to deal with the essential aspects of how both mirror neurons and the Mirror System operate. We would like to stress that this first part *does not intend to be* and *cannot be considered a substitute* for any more in-depth scientific studies on the matter, and we would like to refer our readers to the vast and relevant bibliography currently available, and above all to the excellent work by Professor Rizzolatti and Professor Sinigaglia *Mirrors in the Brain*[2], which we have done our very best to remain as faithful as possible to. Our aim is to introduce those who do not move directly within the scientific world to this extraordinary discovery, and to do so by providing readers with some basic understanding that may enable them to 'break the ice' and subsequently deepen their knowledge alone.

We remain confident that the reader will appreciate our attempt to communicate even the least intuitive concepts contained in these fascinating studies as effectively as we can.

Happy reading!

Matteo Rizzato and Davide Donelli

2 G. Rizzolatti, C. Sinigaglia, *Mirrors in the Brain.*

CHAPTER 1

What are mirror neurons?

Preamble

The discovery of mirror neurons and of the Mirror System in humans is the result of research carried out over the last thirty years by a team of researchers from the University of Parma, Italy, co-ordinated by Professor Giacomo Rizzolatti, with subsequent contributions from other Italian and international scientists.

The awareness that derived from this discovery has turned out to be extremely effective, in that we have now come to consider many aspects of our life from this new perspective.

To reach an overall understanding of the ideas contained in this book, it is necessary to deal with and clarify some basic scientific notions, so as to increase our understanding of what we are talking about and of the way we function.

Once the general outlook of the essential aspects of both mirror neurons and the Mirror System has been mapped out, we will go on to deal with their practical aspects, with a view to highlighting how mirror neurons exert a substantial influence over both the formative and the educational processes of everyone from birth, and equally over the way individuals communicate and interact throughout their lives.

A few concepts

First of all, what is a *neuron*? A neuron is a cell that is specialized in the transmission of impulses from one location to another within our body. Neurons can interact with other neurons and with support cells to form what is known as *nervous tissue,* namely the biological structure that is capable of communicating information from a distance. Just like the wool that is interwoven into a piece of cloth, the nervous tissue is a thick network of neurons where, through the propagation of electrical impulses and the release of certain substances called *neurotransmitters,* communication between different locations within our body is made possible. In turn, nervous tissue is organised into the *nervous system,* which in humans is usually described as made up of two parts: a *central nervous system,* whose components, the brain and the spinal cord, are carefully protected by the cranium and by the spinal column; and a *peripheral nervous system,* which consists of ganglia, plexuses and nerves that branch out across the whole body. Imagine a large country, with large, small and extremely small towns, and just one capital city: they need roads to make sure that communication takes place between them, and somehow they all need to be able to communicate with the capital. In the same way the peripheral nervous system links all the 'towns' in our body (organs, skin, senses, muscles, bones, etc.) with the capital, represented by the central nervous system.

The main characteristic of neurons is their *electrical excitability,* i.e. their capacity to generate an electrical impulse in response to a stimulus; this impulse (known as *action potential*) is propagated throughout the entire neuron, thus transmitting a unity of information from one end to the other. The number of transmitted impulses within a specified time period determines the intensity of the message: if I receive a weak stimulus on my cheek, the tactile neurons which are located on the skin transmit a few impulses per second; if however the stimulus received is strong, the neurons transmit many impulses per second. In both cases this happens according to the same process, that is to say as a consequence of a tactile stimulus.

This excitability lies at the basis of the communication mechanism that exists between neurons: but how does it manifest in a detailed manner? To understand this, we need to improve our knowledge of the common structure of these extraordinary cells, and to this end we will now go into some detail and highlight their most essential features.

Neurons are made up of a *cell body*, an *axon* and several *dendrites* (*Fig. 1*):

- The *cell body* is the central territory of the neuron and contains all the structures that are indispensable both to the life of the cell and to the correct performance of its functions.
- The *axon* is a long, thin projection, which departs from the cell body and can be very long when compared with the size of the cell body. It is characterised by a terminal that branches into 'buttons', which come into contact with either other neurons, or with other types of cells. It is the part of the neuron that *transmits* information either in the direction of other neurons or towards those cells that perform specific functions upon receipt of a signal from the neuron (for example, muscle cells).
- The *dendrites* are highly branched projections resem-

> bling the roots of a tree located close to the cell body. They are much shorter than the axon and can either come into contact with the terminal buttons of the axons of other neurons or directly with other neurons, or can even represent the primary sensory terminations (those terminations from which sensory stimuli such as touch, pain, and sight etc. depart). They are the component that *receives* the information that comes either from other neurons or from the environment.

When a neuron is stimulated near the location of one of its dendrites, the cell body becomes excited and produces an electrical impulse that is 'fired'[3] through the axon.

The communication between neurons occurs in the *synapses,* which are areas made up by the terminal buttons of the first neuron, by the dendrites of the second, and by the space that separates them.

Once the electrical impulse has reached the terminal button it causes the release of chemical substances called *neurotransmitters.* These neurotransmitters then spread out throughout the space of the synapse and reach the surface of the destination neuron, where they find specific receptors with which they can combine, just like fitting a key inside a lock. At this stage the receptors, stimulated by the neurotransmitter, can induce the production of a new electrical impulse in the destination neuron, and so on. Through this mechanism, a stimulus can travel from the tip of one's big toe up to the brain, where it can be interpreted as it passes through complex circuits made up of a huge number of neurons.

However, this does not fully account for how some of our extraordinary abilities–such as movement, thoughts,

3 'Fired' is the actual term used by scientists.

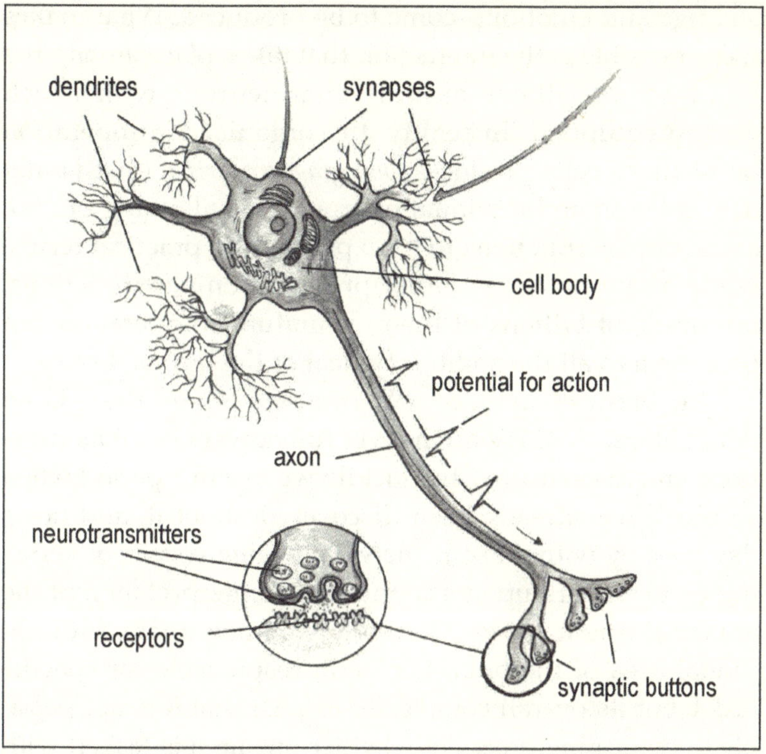

Fig. 1: diagram of the neuron structure. The neuron receives impulses from other neurons and establishes synapses with them. In the upper part of the image we can see two axons from other neurons establishing synapses at the level of the dendrites and of the cell body. The neuron can in turn 'fire', that is to say send out a potential for action, and can propagate it along its axon. In the close-up we can observe in detail a synapse whose neurotransmitters, which are kept within small vesicles inside the synaptic button, are released under the effect of the electrical potential into the intersynaptic space, and subsequently manage to bind with the specific receptors that are located on the destination cell.

feelings and emotions–come to be produced. What makes them possible is the interaction that takes place among the hundreds of billions of individual neurons with which we are equipped. In reality, the organised co-operation of all these cells produces *emerging properties* (that is, not detectable in an individual neuron), thus allowing precise and complex functions to be expressed. In practical terms, while a few neurons cannot produce complex functions, hundreds of billions of them in mutual co-operation can give birth to all the abilities typical of the human brain.

Our brain is an extremely complex organ; there is no doubt about that! We are not yet fully aware of all its functions and mechanisms, but luckily we live in a period when so much has already been discovered about it, and not a day goes by without some new data being collected, allowing us to embark upon a continuous reinterpretation of the amazing way it works. Currently we know that each individual area of the brain is chiefly responsible for specific tasks, but its overall complexity is such that it is not possible to determine precisely whether one area is tasked with just one individual function, or whether it is a member of a 'team' that carries out more complex functions. In fact, it seems that the various parts of the brain, although mainly responsible for managing specific functions, are effectively involved in many other functions. So we are not looking at a simple mechanism, like a motorbike, for instance, which we can take apart, identifying a specific individual function for each part (cylinder, carburettor, transmission, etc.). Rather, we are faced with a complex reality where each part contributes to the functioning of the others.

Having said that, human anatomy has classified the brain (encephalon) into a few main parts, and has identified their main functions (*Fig. 2*):

- the *encephalic trunk,* where the processed information descends first to the spinal cord and subsequently to the body, or moves up from the spinal cord to the upper centres. This is where breathing and cardiac rhythms are set;
- the *cerebellum,* where balance, posture, movement co-ordination and muscular tone are controlled. This area of the brain participates in the emotive and cognitive processes (of thought processing);
- the *diencephalon,* chiefly formed by the thalamus and hypothalamus[4].

  The *thalamus* receives sensory information from both the spinal cord and the encephalic trunk and sends it to the upper parts. The *hypothalamus* is the centre that regulates hunger, thirst, body temperature, arterial pressure, cardiac frequency and sleep-wake rhythms, as well as the working of most of the endocrine glands;
- the *telencephalon,* divided into two hemispheres that are connected in the middle by the corpus callosum. The outer part, the *cerebral cortex,* is folded in on itself in so-called *cerebral convolutions,* separated by grooves. This is the centre where sensory stimuli are perceived; it also controls motor activities and all other superior human functions, including speech and emotions, as well as memory and logical thinking.

The majority of processes typical of both mirror neurons and the Mirror System take place in this part of the

4 To the above-mentioned parts we ought to add the *subthalamus, metathalamus* and *epithalamus*. The epithalamus can be considered similar to the *epiphysis* (or pineal) gland, which is extremely important in setting and adjusting various processes, including the sleep-wake rhythm.

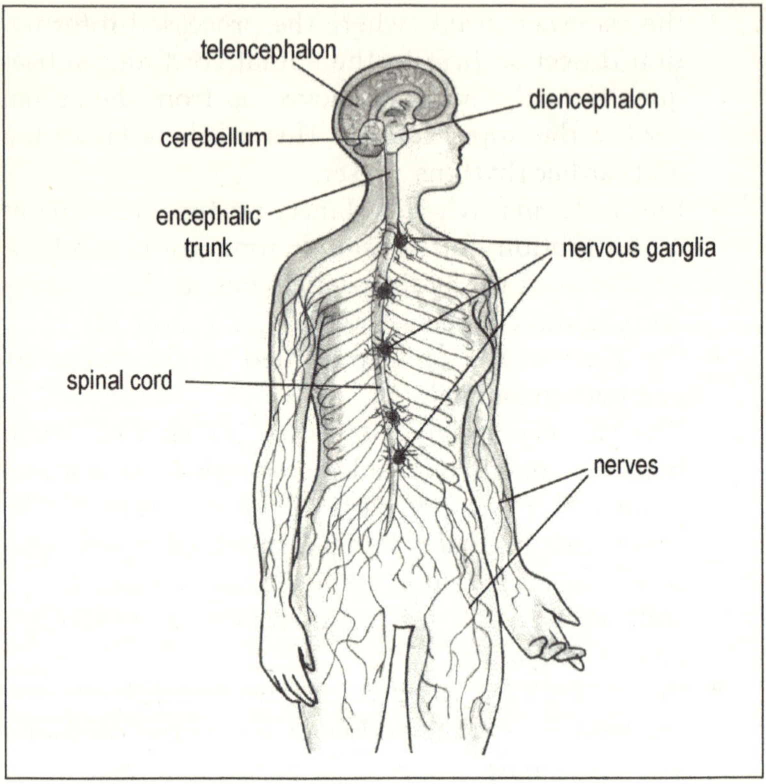

Fig. 2: diagram of the principal parts of the human nervous system.

brain. In particular, the cerebral cortex is the main area of investigation into mirror neurons, which is why we need to examine some of its features in more detail.

At the beginning of the twentieth century, Korbinian Brodmann (1868-1918), a German scientist, classified the cerebral cortex by dividing it topographically into 52 areas (*Fig. 3*), which were identified by analysing the predominant cell typology of each area.

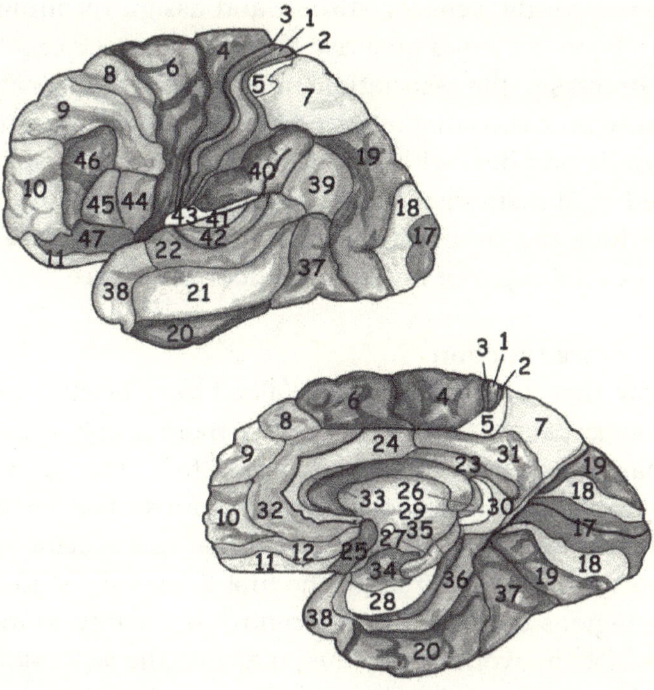

Fig. 3: description of the areas of the cerebral cortex according to Brodmann; each area corresponds to specific functions. As we can see from the numbers, there are 52 areas altogether.

It was hypothesised that each area had a corresponding specific function and at a later stage it became apparent that, as in the case of the whole brain, in the cerebral cortex the different areas also operate in close mutual co-operation. Although a rigidly precise classification of the functions of the various areas is therefore not possible, one or more prevalent functions are nevertheless recognizable.

These areas can be divided into three main categories,

namely *sensory, motor and association areas*: the sensory areas receive the sensory stimuli and assign meaning to them; the motor areas give rise to movements, or regulate their processes; the association areas are the main location for those processes that interpret reality, encode responses to stimuli, and deal with language and emotional aspects, as well as at memorising motor patterns. Finally, they are also where the communicative, imitative, logical and all the so-called superior human functions take place.

The way we function

Now that we have explored (albeit very briefly) these basic concepts, we can begin to enter more deeply into the mechanisms of our brain that we need to be familiar with if we want to begin to understand both mirror neurons and the Mirror System. It must be noted that this specific type of neuron was discovered for the first time while studying those regions of the brain that control the ability to move and which, by working together, make up the *motor system*. It is therefore useful to know how our motor behaviour originates, and how our understanding of it came to be modified as a consequence of the research studies conducted by the team from the University of Parma.

Traditionally our movements are described as the outcome of the action of three main units, located in the cerebral cortex, namely the sensory areas, some association areas, and the primary and secondary motor areas. According to this model, each unit represents a processing 'box', and movement is the result of the flow of information that passes from the first to the second box, from the second to the third, and then from the third to the actual execution. More precisely, these stimuli (which come from outside, and are either of a visual, audito-

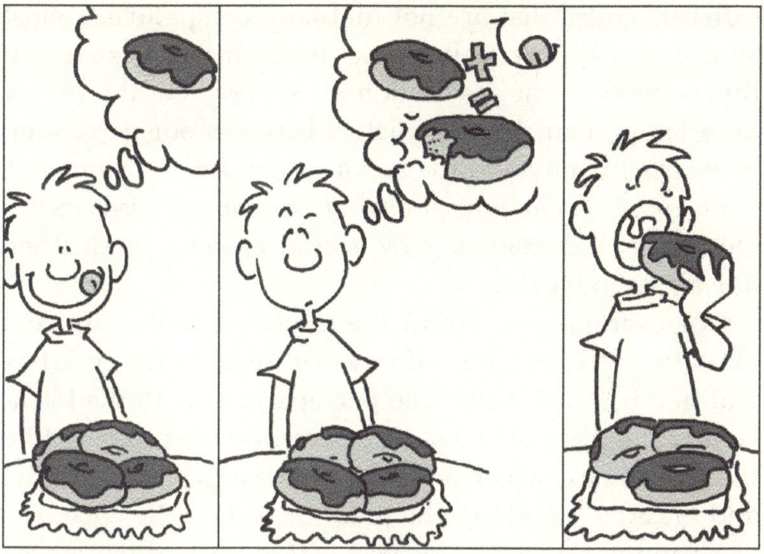

Fig. 4: description of the mass production process. Our character sees the stimulus (a doughnut), processes the received data, and eventually produces an action.

ry, or somatic[5] nature, etc.) are gathered in the sensory areas and transformed into perceptions by association areas, after which other association areas create a motor response to them. Finally the body, upon instructions from the motor areas, carries out the movements.

According to this model, our brain then produces some movement courtesy of a 'I perceive–process–execute' type of process, which is the result of the workings of the three sensory, association and motor units (*Fig. 4*): each of these plays a specific role and operates differently from the others, and the information is processed on the basis of

5 That is touch, pressure, temperature, pain, itch, proprioception and muscle tension.

different codes that are not mutually compatible, almost as if each of these units spoke its own language. From this viewpoint, the association areas carry out the role of 'translators', namely of mediators between our perception of external reality and the act of responding *by translating the meaning of our perceptions into meaningful movements.* Our brain, therefore, acts by a kind of mass production, like an assembly line.

For example, we are in the kitchen and we notice a glass full of water: the information reaches the first box and in our mind creates the perception of both the kitchen and the glass of water; this perception is processed by the second box, which adds the information 'I am thirsty' and encodes 'drinking the glass of water'; the encoding of 'drinking the glass of water' is then carried out by the third box, which executes the body's movements.

This descriptive model of our motor behaviour was suggested by experimental observation of the neuronal activity within the regions where the three 'boxes' are located. Initially it actually looked as if the neurons only became active in connection with their specific function, i.e. the motor area neurons would activate in connection with movements (motor neurons), the sensory area neurons in connection with perceptions (sensory neurons), and those pertaining to the association areas in connection with processing (associative neurons). Recently, however, it has been discovered that it is not as simple as that: in some association areas there are actually some neurons that become active both during data processing, as well as in conjunction with movement, and they can therefore truly be defined as motor neurons. This conflicts with the prior interpretation, and in the light of this discovery,

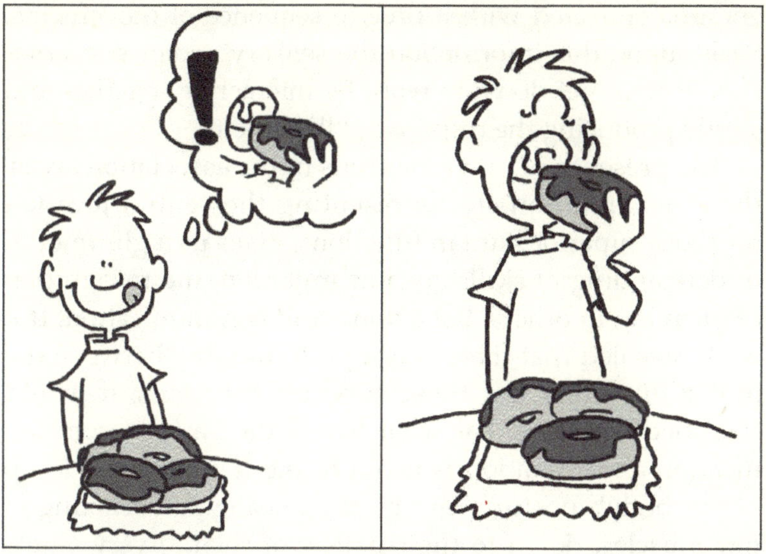

Fig. 5: illustration of parallel processing. At the sight of a stimulus (a doughnut), both associative and motor areas operate simultaneously to produce an immediate response and thus carry out the action of eating.

the motor behaviour pattern has had to be revised: it is no longer thought of as a form of mass production (I perceive–process–execute), but rather as a parallel interaction between various areas, through a common language composed of special neurons that are capable of responding to more than one type of stimulus.

If there is, therefore, a typology of neurons that can drive the outcome of perceptions towards a common format, then the different areas can operate in parallel, dynamically configuring their responses ('in real time') to the surrounding reality (*Fig. 5*).

To recap: when I observe a glass of water, certain specific neurons become active inside me. Whilst some of them are closely related to the object called "glass of water", others are connected with a precise sequence of movements. Based upon this information the sensory, motor and associative areas get down to work by interacting together and jointly producing the response "I'll drink it".

The presence of motor neurons in the association areas, the latter traditionally representing the central location for those superior human functions, gives us a glimmer of understanding of skills such as imitation, the recognition of meaning in others' behaviour, and communication. If it were revealed that there was a profound link between the motor functions and these superior functions, it would then become clear that what lies at the basis of communication and imitation is actually the language made up of our body's posture, and by the tensing and relaxing of our muscles, down to the smallest of them. Every single movement carries some meaning for me, and for others too. In this respect we ought to mention Desmond Morris' research, which highlighted the great importance of the countless gestures that we make, or Paul Ekman's studies of facial microexpressions, which provide even more detailed understanding[6].

Function, not form

It is easy to believe that gestures are coded in series, as a robot would perform in a factory: to move an object, you extend the mechanical arm until it reaches point A, then grab the pliers, then flex the mechanical arm, then move yourself up until you reach point B, then extend the mechanical arm, then open the pliers, and so on and so forth.

Our brain operates differently (thank goodness!), as if both the gesture in its entirety and its objective were

6 Cf. P. Ekman, *Emotions Revealed: Understanding Faces and Feelings*, Orion, 2004.

prefigured inside the brain from the very outset, and both remain very clear and focussed throughout the execution. If you wanted to make one click with your mouse, your brain would encode each single relevant movement at the same time, i.e. extend the arm, squeeze the fingers, move the wrist and finally click by using your index finger. All these movements would be encoded right from the start, and executed in the correct order.

In this respect the team headed by Professor Rizzolatti has discovered a very important characteristic that pertains to those neurons located in a specific area of the cerebral cortex, the *premotor area*: they 'encode', meaning that they programme the information required for executing complex actions with a precise purpose, but they do not do it in the case of basic, individual and specific movements (such as a simple stretch of the forearm). There are therefore some 'specialized' neurons that correspond to complex actions with very specific goals, and these become selectively active depending on their *function*: 'grab' neurons, 'move' neurons, 'pull' neurons, 'squeeze' neurons, etc.

For example, if I grab hold of my wrist, in the premotor area a specific population of neurons becomes activated; if I grab a glass, a *different* neuron population is activated, although the movement is similar to the first one (it is still grabbing, but it is grabbing different items for different purposes). Again, if I flex my fingers to play a guitar, specific neurons are activated, but if I bend my fingers to scratch myself, *other* neurons are activated instead. A very specific population of neurons becomes activated for each specific goal-directed action (namely a gesture with a purpose, such as picking up a glass of water). These 'leader' neurons that encode complete goal-directed actions lead us to understand that it is possible simultaneously to encode every single movement that is required to carry out a complex action: it is thanks to them that all the different neuronal populations involved in the encoding of basic movements can manage to co-ordinate themselves and act in the correct sequential order.

The understanding of this dynamic was an extraordinary event, as it radically alters how we interpret the mechanisms that lie at the basis of our movements. The key point guiding how our actions are encoded is therefore not their *form,* but their *function,* their purpose! Irrespective of the movements that I have to make, what actually matters is whether I need to grab something or somebody or myself, and then move it, damage it, protect it, hold it, etc. Hence it does not matter a great deal whether I move my arm to the right or to the left, whether I rotate my wrist, close my hand, etc.; what matters is *what I want to do,* what my objective is.

Let us imagine that I want to pick up a piece of chocolate that is lying on a table. My brain does not operate in terms of 'extend your arm from here to there, then close your fingers once they are close to the chocolate, then exert some strength, then bend your arm, etc.', but rather in terms of '*pick up* the chocolate', and on the basis of this objective it directs all the movements needed to perform the action. In fact, while we are picking up the chocolate, some areas in our cerebral cortex hold the constant prefiguration of our purpose, that is to say 'pick up the object'. From the very outset those specific motor areas that are required to carry out the action (i.e. reach the chocolate, grab it, bring it to your mouth, etc.) are activated, and the individual movements are executed in the correct order and a continuous flow, on the basis of spatial references.

Visual motor neurons

Let us move a step closer to becoming acquainted with our friends, the mirror neurons. Research conducted by Professor Rizzolatti and his team has revealed that one part of those selective 'leader-neurons' (namely the ones that become activated in conjunction with a specific action) also responds to specific *visual* stimuli: they can also become activated when we see something. These neurons are said to possess some *visual motor* characteristics; in other words, they possess some properties that allow them to respond to specific sight-originated stimuli, and some motor properties that cause them to respond to the performing of an action. What does all this mean?

Practically speaking, these neurons become activated both in conjunction with the execution of an action and at the sight of certain objects: in particular they become activated when we carry out the action that they are encoding (such as 'grabbing', for instance), or when we observe an object that possesses some specific characteristics. The objects that activate these neurons are those that provide us with an opportunity for interaction, by means of the action encoded by the neurons themselves. In other words, the visual motor neurons are accurately classified as 'leader neurons' (thus there are 'grab' visual motor neurons, 'move' visual motor neurons, and so on), and the difference lies in that, in addition to being activated when their specific action is being carried out, they are also activated when we observe an object that we could use through that particular action.

For instance, if I were to grab the pen that is lying on the table, some specific visual motor neurons would be activated, and if I were to observe the same pen lying on the table, the *same* visual motor neurons would be activated. This is the key to understanding how we interact with the objects that surround us: there are some neurons that link objects with the actions that are compatible with their use. Although a simple observation activates the motor neurons, this does not necessarily mean that the action will be carried out: as a matter of fact, the activation of visual motor neurons in the course of the observation phase remains at the *level of potential*, i.e. that action has not been executed.

Objects? No, hypotheses!

So, how do the recognition of an object and the association of a relevant action occur in detail?

To understand this, we need to introduce a concept known in technical terms as *affordances*[7]: these are the *options* at our disposal when we interact with an object in practical terms. To be more precise, these *affordances* are the interaction opportunities that an object may offer to whoever sees it (*Fig. 6*). The objects that surround us have the most diverse shapes, which offer various interaction opportunities: for example, a cup would offer me three main options for interacting with it, namely body, handle and brim.

Whenever we see an object, this object is 'broken down' into its options in a specific area of the cerebral cortex, and one of the options is selected based upon two factors: the actor's intentions and the 'conceptual' recognition of the object. It must be noted that our intentions come from an area called the prefrontal cortex, whereas the recognition of the meaning of objects takes place in the lower temporal lobe[8].

7 J.J. Gibson, *The ecological approach to visual perception*, Houghton Mifflin, 1979.
8 It is in this area that conceptual meaning is associated with

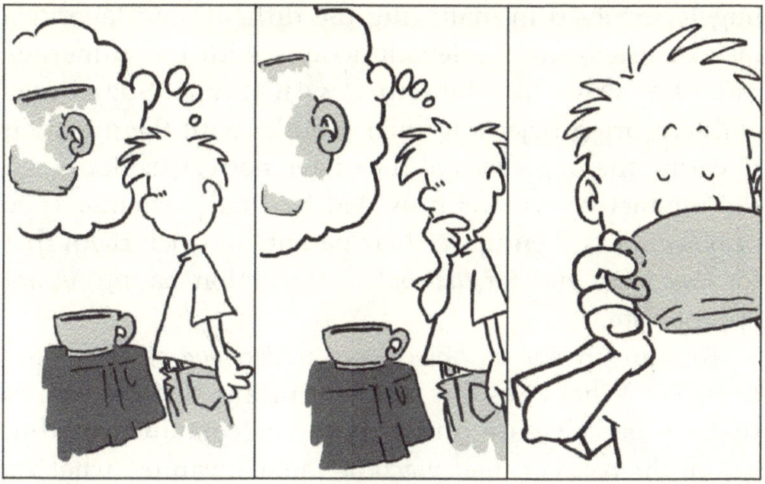

Fig. 6: options for interaction. Our character sees a cup of coffee and immediately in his brain the cup is 'broken down' into those parts that provide an opportunity for interaction, in this case brim, handle and body. Subsequently, by adding the intention, namely drinking the coffee, the brain selects the most appropriate option, i.e. the handle.

Once the meaning of the object has been recognised and we have decided what we intend to do, the selected option is presented to the premotor area, where the relevant action is encoded by virtue of the work carried out by the visual motor neurons.

The type of action that is relevant to a specific option is determined in childhood by motor learning, during which time one or more congruent and effective motor acts are associated with each of the options. This is particularly interesting when we consider how children learn, given that during their early years they are already

the images that we see (for instance, when I see a pencil I recognise it chiefly as a writing tool).

hugely involved in managing the difficult and laborious task of 'associating' relevant actions with the numerous potential ways of interacting with things. Sometimes children bring objects to their mouths with the intention of eating them, given that they have not yet 'explored' all the interactive options provided by that particular type of object. It is then up to their parents to teach them that for *that thing* and for *that option* the action 'eating' is not appropriate.

To sum up, for us objects are *understood* as *hypotheses for action*. What does this mean? It means that the objects that we perceive are understood (i.e. 'contained' within us) on the basis of their *practical* value, meaning 'what we can do' in our interaction with them, rather than on the basis of their meaning. When we are actually engaged in the process of observation, a certain portion of our visual motor neurons is inevitably activated within us, and this connects us directly to the object: it is a relation that has to do with what *we can do* with it.

Action vocabulary

At this juncture we can introduce an idea of paramount importance: the *action vocabulary*[9].

Studies have shown that the premotor area contains various populations of visual motor neurons, each of which encodes for either the oriented action (grabbing, pulling out, and so on) or for its mode of execution (gentle, accurate, strong grip, and so on), or for the time sequence of its movements. Each population represents a 'word' and the population group makes up the action vocabulary; the *sentences* are composed from the word

9 Or vocabulary of acts; Cf. Rizzolatti and Sinigaglia, *Mirrors in the Brain*.

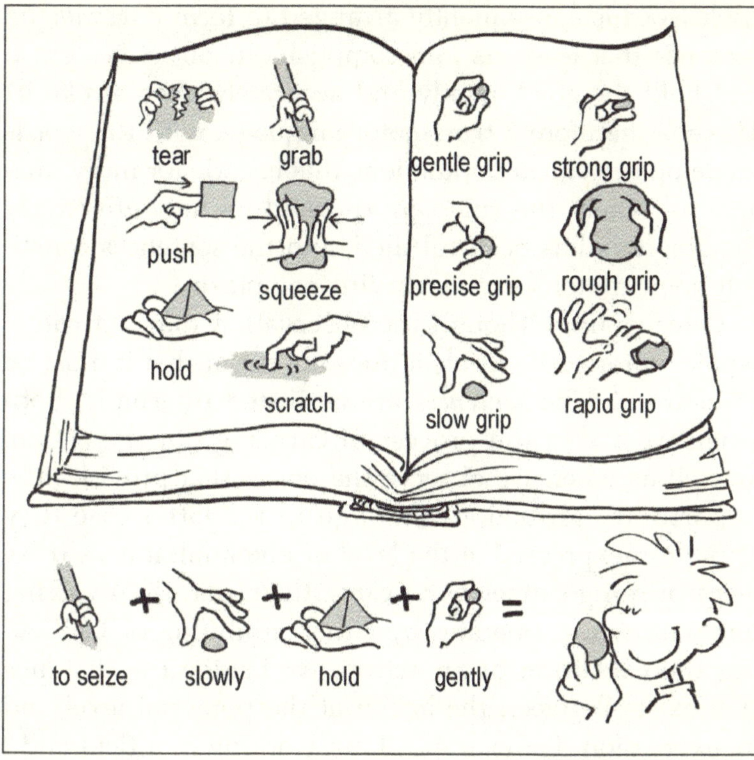

Fig. 7: illustration of the action vocabulary. This area of our brain can be compared to a real dictionary that contains motor words, and the combination of these 'words' gives rise to actions.

combinations and they constitute real actions, ranging from the simplest to the most complex (*Fig. 7*).

Let us imagine a situation where we would like to pick up and stroke a chick: we first observe it, then select the most suitable way to pick it up, after which in our premotor area several words that are consistent with the circumstances become activated: 'grabbing', 'gentle grip', 'accurate grip', 'stroking', 'first grabbing, then stroking'.

Each word is subsequently arranged to form a *meaningful* sentence that leads us to accomplish our objective: 'grasp and hold the chick gently and accurately, then stroke it'. There is therefore a true motor language, with the words made up of neuron populations that encode for individual actions, where the rules are dictated by how effectively the objective has been fulfilled, and the sentences constitute some motor *scenes* of varying complexity.

Once again, although the observation may activate a whole motor scene in us, it does not mean that it must be carried out. The *sentences* are activated internally, both when we are in the process of carrying out the action, as well as when we observe the object that provides the opportunity for action–although in the latter case they remain unexpressed at the level of potential: it is as if we were priming ourselves to carry them out. By involving our will, which operates by either inhibiting or facilitating the execution of an action, we bridge the distance that exists between the action at the potential level and its expression. For example, I am working in a field and I am very thirsty: I see an abundant flow of irrigation water gushing out and the entire scene required for drinking is prefigured within me. However, I know that this is not drinking water, and therefore the motor sentence that encodes for drinking remains at a potential level, without being expressed.

Even at this early stage it is important to specify that when we interact with other living beings–as opposed to objects–the situation changes, especially when emotions are involved. As we will see, it is exactly at this point that we come across the practical application of the discovery of mirror neurons, but for the moment let us proceed in an orderly manner.

Spatial representation

When a certain action has to be carried out, the space around us plays a crucial role, and even more crucial is the way in which our brain describes it. When we look around, the description of space seems a very simple thing to do: there is us, and then there is the environment within which we move. It appears that the environment is static and that we are the ones moving about by using various objects as reference points: if we had to orient ourselves, we would trace some fixed coordinates across the environment as reference points and would then make use of them to define our position.

However, the work conducted by the team from the University of Parma has shown that when we interact with objects, space is not described as a fixed set of coordinates within which we move, but as a *dynamic* and variable system, its coordinates centred around the various parts of our body. The brain therefore does not assign absolute positions to the objects that surround us relative to a hypothetical centre that corresponds to our body; instead it perceives them as *action hypotheses* circumscribed within a *relative* space. This space is described on the basis of the relationships that exist between the parts of our body, the perceived object and what we can do with the latter. Essentially, we constantly redefine our perception of space according to what we *can* do and *consider* doing with the objects that are contained within it. This constant redefinition makes our description of space a relative one, and this is easy to demonstrate. For us the concepts of *near* and *far* are completely relative, depending on the type of action that we considering. If I cross the road and there is a car approaching at a very high speed, the car will seem to be *near* me when it reaches a distance

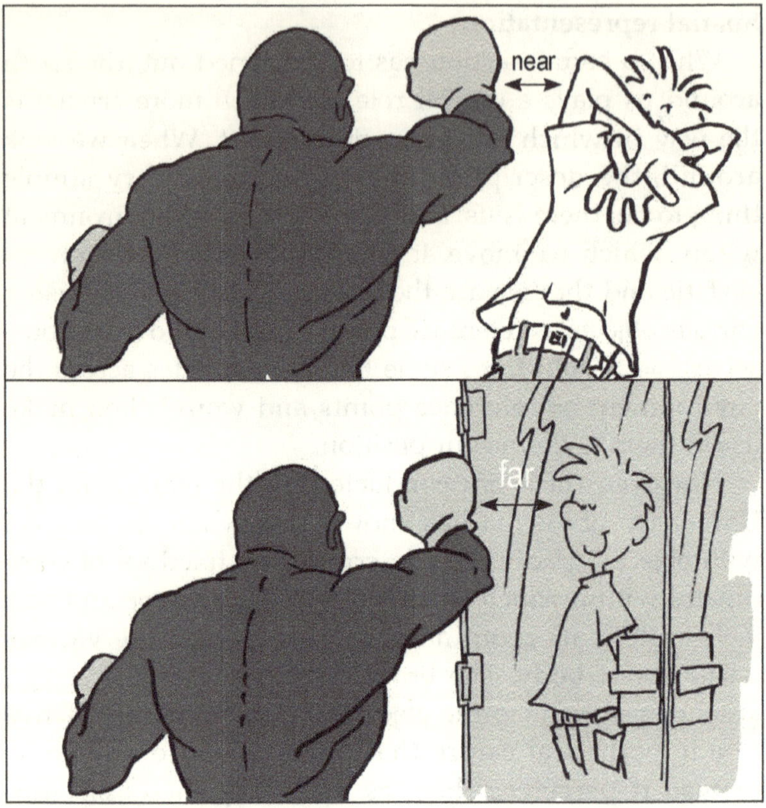

Fig. 8: relativity of spatial representation.

of ten yards, whereas if I need to get to my car that is parked at exactly the same distance, it will seem farther away than the one in the speeding car example (*Fig. 8*).

Similarly, other aspects of special representation, such as *reachable* or *unreachable, big* or *small, fast* or *slow, straight* or *bent* and so on are equally relative, as they are susceptible to the constant redefinition of space.

Sometimes, however, it is our body's limits that are

redefined, such as the moment when we pick up an object to carry out an action from a distance. If, for instance, I use a long spoon to stir some soup, the spoon becomes the new limit, the extension of my body. If you think about it, each time we stir the contents of the pot we do not have to calculate the distance, given that it has become *automatic,* as if our arm itself had become extended.

This is how actions become the pivotal point in defining both our space and our motor behaviour: first, what we perceive as space is what we *can* do and *consider doing* with whatever surrounds us, just like all surrounding objects are first of all perceived as action hypotheses. This forces us to observe once again how actions are a priority for our brain.

Mirror neurons

We have already seen how our brains contain neuron populations that possess the ability to become active both in response to a motor act and to the visual stimuli connected with that particular motor act: these are called *canonical neurons*. The studies conducted by Rizzolatti and Gentilucci, and subsequently by Murata and his colleagues[10], have highlighted that canonical neurons are not the only neurons that possess visual motor abilities: there are in fact populations of neurons that become active when a movement is made, as well as when *someone else is observed* making a similar movement, and these are called *mirror neurons* (*Fig. 9*). What are the distinguishing features of mirror vis-a-vis canonical neurons? The answer lies in their visual properties, that is to say the quality of the response that a neuron gives to a specific typology of visual stimulation. Mirror neurons do not become active when observing objects with which they could potentially

10 Cf. bibliography.

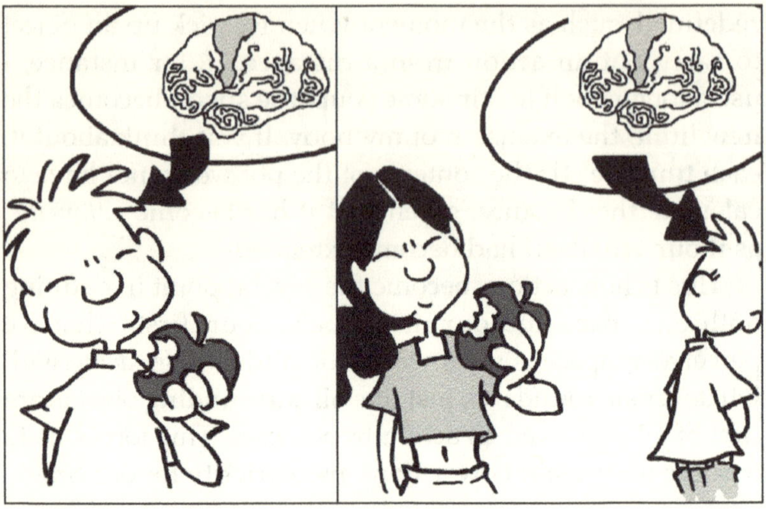

Fig. 9: mirror neuron activation. The boy watches the girl bite the apple, and the same mirror neurons that would activate if he were the one biting the apple become active in his brain.

interact, but in conjunction with the actions that are carried out by another person, *especially* if these actions entail interacting with an object.

Basically when we observe somebody doing something, at the level of neuronal activation it is tantamount to us doing it ourselves; or rather, we *prepare ourselves* to do it, and therefore we can *be closer to understanding what others perceive when they are in the process of doing it.*

As with canonical neurons, all the various populations of mirror neurons represent an action vocabulary, where each word corresponds to an action. Therefore, there are populations of mirror-grab neurons, mirror-reach neurons, mirror-turn neurons and so forth. This is of paramount importance in that it is actually on the basis of known 'motor words' that we can build up a common lan-

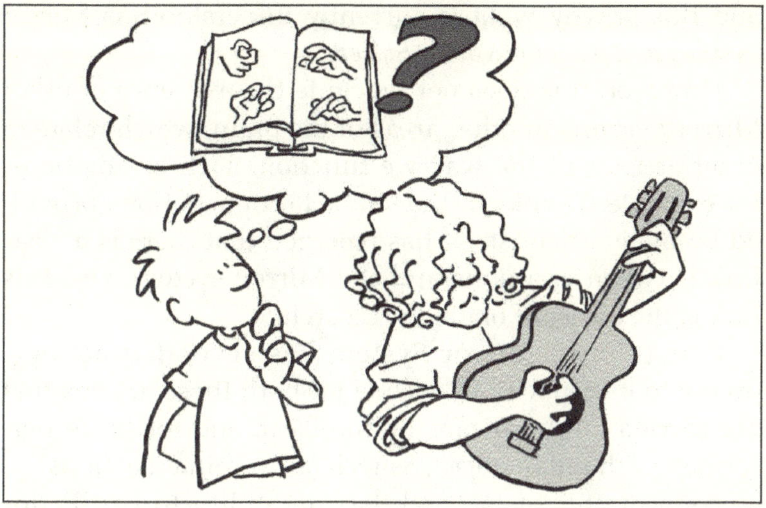

Fig. 10: our young man watches the guitarist play, but his motor vocabulary does not yet contain suitable 'words' that would allow him to accurately identify the movements that the other is making.

guage that allows us to understand other people's actions.

This is why, when we observe actions made up of movements that are not part of our vocabulary, we are not able to understand the meaning of the action observed, or at least not entirely, given that we would only be able to understand it in accordance with the terminology that is contained in our own vocabulary. If at my first guitar lesson I watch my teacher play, I understand the action in terms of 'move the pick and press the strings using the fingers', but what still eludes me is the entire sequence of detailed movements that enable him to create such a wonderful melody (*Fig. 10*).

In humans, mirror neurons as a whole make up what is defined as the *Mirror System*. The studies conducted to date have focused primarily on motor mirror neurons, and this is why what is currently understood as Mirror System is the *Motor Mirror System.*

However, this does not preclude the existence of other Mirror Systems in other areas of the brain, which relate to other aspects of the way we function, such as emotions, for example. Thanks to the valuable contributions provided by many scientists, it has emerged that there is a clear link between emotions and the Mirror System, and this link is the object of ongoing research[11].

Our (Motor) Mirror System has several functions, owing to its capacity to encode for both those actions that are carried out by means of an object, and for those performed without an object, as well as for mimed actions.

As a matter of fact, whilst the ability to codify for actions that include objects is developed among monkeys too, the ability to codify for actions without objects, or for mimed actions (such as imitating the use of a specific tool even though the tool may be missing) is a distinguishing feature that characterises humans alone. In short, humans can–if they so wish–pretend to use an "imaginary" object that does not exist, such as pretending to pick up the telephone, whereas monkeys do not have the ability to do it.

The monkeys' mirror system, for instance, is capable of codifying only a few actions without objects, namely those that have a communicative function (showing one's teeth, pouting one's lips, etc.). The mirror system in humans, however, can codify a huge amount of actions of this type and our communicative abilities are proof of it. Even very young children–when learning how to do something–must first of all imitate the action, adopt it as a model and then repeat it until they make it theirs: humans learn by imitating other humans.

11 Rizzolatti and Sinigaglia, *Mirrors in the Brain*, Ch. 7.

The function of mirror neurons

What is the exact function of mirror neurons? The studies by Rizzolatti and his team from the University of Parma have revealed that mirror neurons: *"lie at the heart of the recognition and understanding of the meaning of others' actions"*. Through the observation of another person's actions, mirror neurons enable us to understand their meaning immediately. In fact, while we observe someone carrying out an action, a selection process takes place among the 'motor words' contained in our vocabulary, until those corresponding to what we are observing have been located. What is happening at a neuronal level is that among the populations of mirror neurons those that most resonate with what is being observed become most intensely activated.

In our cerebral cortex what is evoked, so to speak, is a *potential action* that corresponds to the action that is being observed. Obviously this potential action is not expressed by our body, but in our cerebral cortex it is 'as if' we were carrying it out! As we have seen, for a potential action to be stimulated to the point of being executed, intention must be present. The simple evocation in us of the observed action allows the instantaneous comprehension of its *practical* meaning, and it is as if we really 'contained' the action itself, as if we were 'carrying it out without doing it', being aware both of its essence and function.

We could see it in the following terms: it is as if one part of our cerebral cortex had the ability to come into resonance with the observed actions. What does that mean? Resonance is a physical phenomenon, whereby if an object has a specific oscillation frequency and receives waves in phase[12] and

12 Two waves or periodic movements with the same frequency are considered to be in phase when their initial impulses occur at the very same time. When I push a child on a swing, my

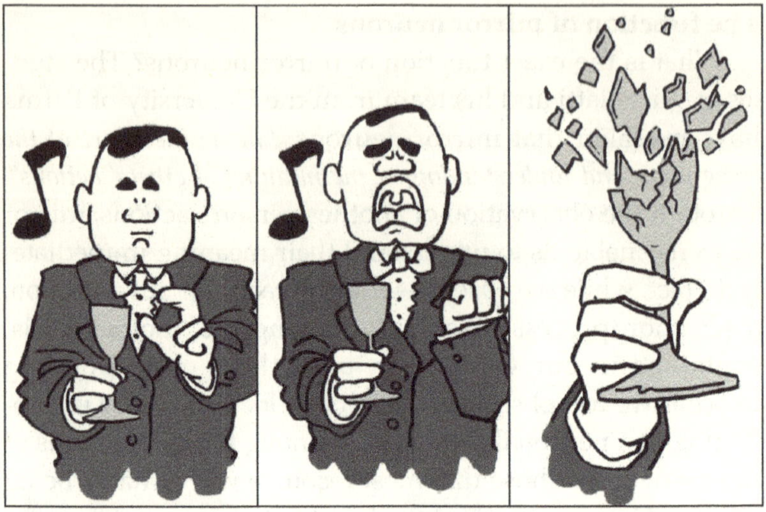

Fig. 11: resonance. Enrico Caruso taps the glass to listen to the note that is produced by the vibration. He then sings an identical note, with exactly the same frequency and, due to the resonance and the power of his voice, he smashes the glass.

with the same frequency, it then absorbs energy.

This is the principle whereby the great Caruso would break crystal glasses when singing a note at precisely the same frequency that made it come into resonance with the glass (*Fig. 11*).

To give another example, if I have two guitars in the same room and I play the fourth string of one of them, the fourth string of the other will begin to vibrate in resonance. Similarly, when I observe another person carrying out an action and my Mirror System comes into resonance with

pushing is normally in phase with the oscillations of the swing, thus perpetuating the movement. If I started pushing out of phase, the swing would either come to a halt, or its oscillations would decrease.

it, this activates in me everything that relates to this action and its purpose.

Intention

Actions can be the result of combining a number of simple movements, as in the example of playing the violin: the individual movements of the left and right hands are linked together to form the action of playing. This sequence consists of a series of activations of neuronal populations that are specifically related to individual movements. These movements, when expressed in a particular sequential order, produce the desired action. We are talking about a *motor sentence*, the result of the well-ordered sequence of a number of *words* contained in one's vocabulary, and this is what our Mirror System recognises, from the very outset, when observing the actions of another person.

Let us now review the selection process that brings us to the recognition of the meaning contained in someone else's actions.

When the intention of an action that has been observed has not yet been clearly identified, our Mirror System simultaneously activates a number of neuronal populations, those 'motor words' of ours that correspond to either individual movements, or to execution modes. From these, both those compatible with what we are observing and those that are not are equally activated. This is because the choice of the 'word' that most *resonates* with the observations has not yet been made. As this selection gradually takes place, those 'words' that are most compatible with what we are observing are gradually activated with increasing intensity from within these populations (*Fig. 12*).

I see a man sitting at a table on top of which lies an

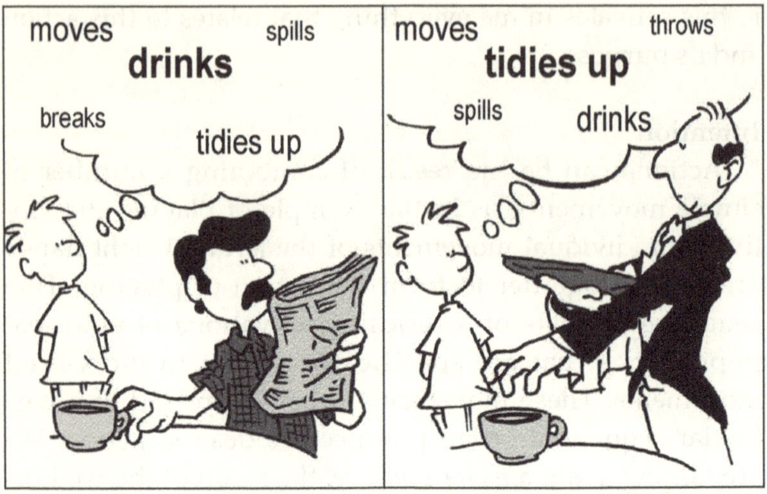

Fig. 12: recognition of the intention. Through the observation of either the man reading the paper or the waiter, in our character's brain a selection process takes place as regards the potential intentions of these two people. The selection is carried out on the basis of the intention which most resonates with the scene that is being observed. In the first panel the hand of the man who prefigures grabbing the cup's handle is effectively directing the selection towards drinking, whereas the hand of the waiter who prefigures seizing the body of the cup is directing it towards tidying up.

object. I observe the man prefiguring[13] how to pick up the object and thereby my Mirror System immediately

13 In this particular context the term 'prefiguring' can have different meanings. It can indicate the form that a movement takes in relation to its goal, in a synergistic relationship with its achievement: for instance, the form that a hand takes when it wishes to stroke a face and when, just before doing so, it 'prefigures' the face that it will touch. Alternatively it may indicate the prefiguring of an action in the brain, when all the neuronal populations that correspond to a specific complete action become activated, irrespective of whether the action is then carried out or not. In this respect, the action is actually 'figured out in advance' of being carried out.

activates various (motor) 'terms', such as *grabbing, pushing, touching slightly, vigorously, accurately.* Given however that the action that is about to be performed has not yet been specified–in the sense that its intention has not been recognised–the Mirror System activates all the motor 'terms' which, according to our motor knowledge, could end up making up the action that I am in the process of observing.

Among these 'words', those that are most intensely activated are those *most* suitable for the circumstances. As I gradually observe other people's actions and collect data, my Mirror System further specifies the selection of the potential motor words, increasingly directing itself towards the correct 'motor sentence'. If I notice that the mouth of the man sitting at the table is beginning to open slightly, my Mirror System promptly orients itself towards an act of eating.

The recognition of the intention of an action is based upon a common motor language, which means that I recognise when, thanks to the Mirror System, I myself potentially experience the very action that I am observing. It is as if a motor 'word' was communicated to me, which entered me and made me 'ready' for that particular action, and therefore capable of understanding it. This recognition of intention goes beyond interpretation, in that it does not occur in that part of the brain that normally makes up 'stories' by interpolating the data gathered from the senses with elements from memory, or of a cultural, educational or experiential nature, and so forth[14], but is strictly linked to the practical dimension, the archetype of action, that is to say, to the achievement of a practical objective, such as eating, sniffing, protecting oneself, moving about and so

14 Cf. *Methods in Mind,* M. Gazzaniga, C. Senior, T. Russel (eds.), MIT Press, 2006.

on. It follows therefore that in this recognition of the intentions of other people's actions, there is no involvement of interpretative elements, and what is involved instead are motor elements (or 'words'), which have been acquired through motor learning. When another person carries out an action, I know how to recognise his or her intention on the basis of the motor data that I am observing (so long as I am familiar with the motor words that the other is using, as we shall see later), and as the action progressively unfolds, I gather data that will allow me to prefigure its purpose. At the beginning I am not in possession of any data and all options, meaning the motor words, are equivalent. I then observe the hand of the person prefiguring a particular type of grip and I therefore only select the most likely options/motor words. Finally, I notice a precise prefiguration of the hand, and thus the Mirror System selects only one word, that which is most compatible and which therefore best corresponds to the intention this allows me to prefigure, and therefore understand and recognise the action, even before it is fully executed (*Fig. 13*).

When the Mirror System recognises the intention of the other's action, based on the data received from both motor knowledge and circumstances, then the entire action is configured within it at the level of potential, given that all the required specific neuronal populations (motor words) have been activated in the correct sequence (sentence). This is a dynamic process, which is constantly renewed through the gathering of new data through observation, and therefore our Mirror System automatically redefines and reinterprets the actions that it observes, thus producing an increasingly clear and defined real time understanding of the action observed. It is really extraordinary that facial micromovements alone

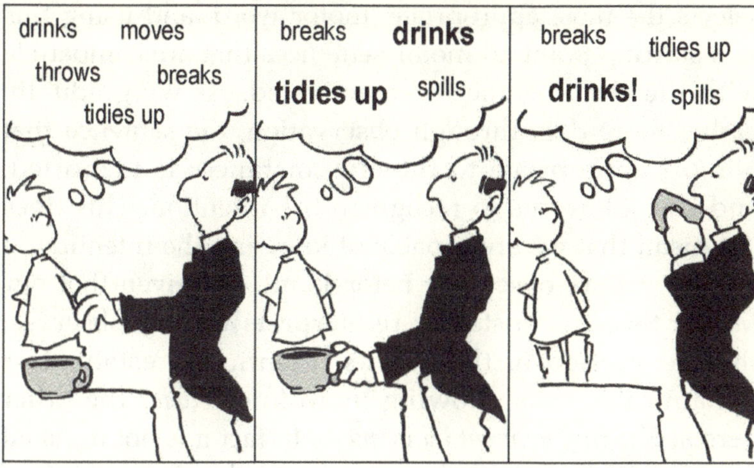

Fig. 13: recognition of the intention. As our character gradually gathers data through observing the waiter (an example chosen to maintain narrative continuity with Figure 12, although we could have chosen any other context), he is increasingly able to recognise the intention. In the second panel we can already see how the observation of the waiter taking hold of the handle directs the selection towards drinking, while in the third panel both the slight opening of the mouth and bringing the cup closer definitely direct the selection towards the intention of drinking the coffee.

(and there are so many of them) are enough to make us totally redefine our interpretation of another's action[15].

The same holds true for the interpretations that others give to our actions: even the smallest detail *enters* and activates different neuronal populations and thus give rise to different interpretations.

What are you doing?

To recap, when the Mirror System comes into resonance with an action carried out by another person, it

15 Cf. *Emotions Revealed: Understanding Faces and Feelings.*

selects the most appropriate 'motor word' and using this as a starting point all motor sentences that are compatible with the circumstances are activated. As we gradually gather more data through observation, the sentence that is most appropriate to the circumstances is identified, and this allows us to recognise the intention. This does not mean that we are capable of knowing the intention of anyone we are observing beforehand, but given that our Mirror System constantly reinterprets what it observes, the recognition of the other's intention is established dynamically, thus allowing us to know *what* the other person *is doing, moment by moment.* In fact it is not unusual to observe somebody changing his or her intention half way through an action. I see someone about to insert a coin into a coffee vending machine, only to stop and put the coin back in his pocket. Alternatively, I see a woman extending her hand towards some tempting pastry, only to stop herself and quickly withdraw it (*Fig. 14*).

Its ability to instantaneously redefine and reinterpret the observed action allows our Mirror System to recognise that the person's intentions have changed.

Once I have recognised the intention of the action that I have observed, I can recall all the motor words that are required to understand and reproduce said action.

What is more, when we know *what* the other *is doing,* our Mirror System recalls the entire motor sentence required to reproduce the action, even with scenes of a complex nature.

Furthermore, if the intention is easily recognizable, the entire sequence of movements required to perform the action is evoked within me from the very beginning, even if I do not see it all. For instance, if I see a man in a coffee bar moving his hand towards a cup of coffee, but then I

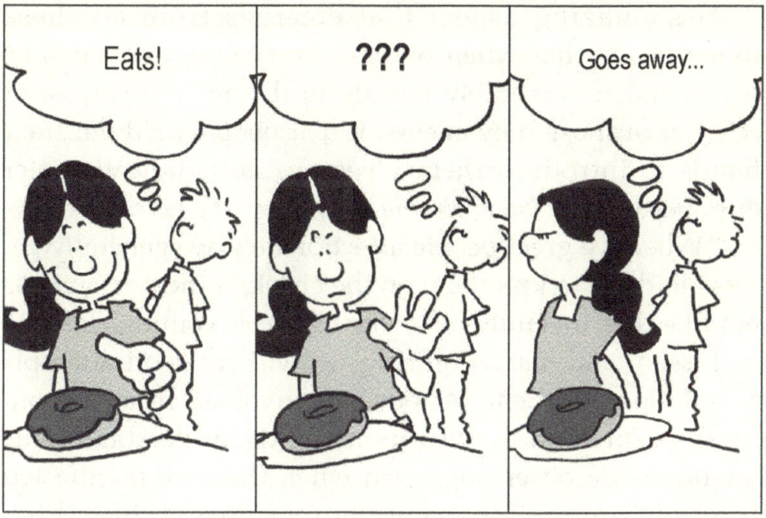

Fig. 14: change of intention. The boy observes the girl stretching out her hand and prefiguring picking up the doughnut: he therefore recognises her intention to eat. Subsequently the girl removes her hand, thus invalidating the intention to eat. The mirror system manages to adjust itself in real time and immediately recognises the new intention.

immediately close my eyes, I will still be aware of what he is doing and be able to reproduce the whole action within me, because I immediately recognised his intention (to drink the coffee). Recognizing the intention equates to possessing within oneself at the level of potential the whole sequence of motor words required for picking up the cup and drinking the coffee.

This is the why, if I decide to perform the same action I observed, the sequence of movements required to carry it out is already prefigured within me, so long as my vocabulary contains the 'suitable words' that correspond to the individual movements or modalities, and which correspond to the individual movements, or modes of execution.

The amazing aspect that emerges from all these dynamics is that when others observe our movements, they manage incredibly rapidly to deduce the *purpose or objective* of those movements. When people hold out their hands to introduce themselves, we automatically offer ours because *we know already* why they are holding theirs out. When we greet people affectionately, we generally get close to them to kiss them on the cheek; if the person does not like this, instantly he or she *will avoid* coming closer to be kissed, and just as quickly we will cease all attempts to get close to them. Whoever is involved in a communicative interaction with us instantly understands our intentions by observing, even when they are manifested through almost imperceptible movements. Just think how many considerations arise each day in relation to the actions that we observe in others, and those that others observe in us! How much do these actions say about us? How much do others understand what we are about to do? And above all, how much do our thoughts or beliefs modify such actions? And is this perceived? We are transparent in almost everything, and our actions also make our intentions explicit.

I cannot see? In that case I will listen!

Everything that we have discussed so far in relation to the Mirror System is not only applicable to what we see, but also to what we *hear*. The various neuronal populations include *bimodal* neurons capable of responding to auditory, as well as visual, stimuli.

These neurons can also be found among mirror neurons, and this is one way for us to recognise and understand someone else's actions, simply on the basis of the sounds that we can hear.

Just as in the case of mirror neurons that respond to visual stimuli, bimodal neurons for the auditory aspect belong to neuronal populations that encode for specific actions and therefore make up the 'words' of a motor vocabulary.

This is one reason whereby we can evoke a potential action within ourselves, simply by virtue of an auditory stimulus: if I am happily walking down the street and at some point I hear the sound of a man running behind me, immediately the potential action of running is configured within me and, if I consider it necessary, the action can be approved and then carried out by my body.

Understanding

By now it is clear to us that understanding others' motor actions is not a cognitive process–that is to say it is not the result of 'thinking', which requires some type of processing followed by a response–but is an immediate and concrete evocation within us of the very essence of what we are observing. This effectively ensures that we are equipped with a 'common language' of motor actions that facilitates the immediate understanding of intentions, where by understanding we are not referring to an abstract concept but to something that 'contains within itself' the action and its purpose. To be even more precise, Professor Rizzolatti describes this understanding of intentions as: "depending upon the automatic selection of strategies of action which, on the basis of our wealth of motor knowledge, each time turn out to be those most compatible with the observed scenario"[16].

This is why: "as soon as we see someone carrying out an action or a chain of actions, then whether that someone

16 G. Rizzolatti, C. Sinigaglia, *Mirrors in the Brain,* p. 127.

likes it or not, his movements immediately acquire significance for us. Obviously, the same applies to the opposite situation: every one of our actions immediately takes on meaning for those observing those actions. Possession of the MNS (mirror neuron system) and the selectivity of their responses thus determine a space of shared action, within which each act, each chain of actions, whether they be executed by us immediately appears to be inscribed and *comprehended* without such operations requiring an explicit and deliberate cognitive operation"[17].

This *space of shared action* is a key point for understanding the importance of our contact with others, the possibilities and *responsibilities* that this entails, irrespective of the direction in which our will is oriented.

We now know for a fact that whenever we find ourselves in a *space of shared* action, *we are inside what the other is doing* and conversely the other is inside what we are doing. If we reflect on this for a moment, this means that we communicate our intentions constantly and inevitably, and others cannot help but experience them within themselves. By reproducing what I do within themselves, whether they like it or not, others reflect what I am doing, just like standing in front of a mirror.

Vocabulary differences

Within this space of shared action, it should be noted how some potential differences of vocabulary can be of great importance.

As we have seen, the vocabulary of the Mirror System is the instrument that enables us to translate what we observe into a real action or chain of potential actions within ourselves. When there are discrepancies between

17 Ibid. (our italics).

the vocabularies of the individuals present within the space of shared action, it is possible that they do not share a full understanding of the observed action. In fact, if I am observing my horse is neighing, the Mirror System does not become activated in me, because my human vocabulary does not contain the 'words' required to understand the meaning of an action that belongs solely to the animal world.

On the other hand, if I observe my horse eating, the Mirror System will become active in me, because I possess terms of reference with regard to the action of eating. In any case, it will be activated at a significantly lower level than for any possible observation of one of my own kind, because inevitably our vocabulary contains more 'human words' than 'equine words'.

This also occurs at a different level, between human beings, whenever vocabulary differences might be caused by some different motor knowledge. A perfect example is that of a dancer and of a beginner when they both observe a ballet teacher (*Fig. 15*). The former will experience a significant activation of the Mirror System, because by virtue of his previous effort (years of training) he has enriched his vocabulary of such actions, and has acquired a motor knowledge that enables him to fully appreciate what he is observing. The beginner, on the other hand, will experience a weak activation of the Mirror System, and he will only understand those actions contained within the motor sequence executed by the teacher that he is capable of retaining, based upon his limited knowledge of ballet. Each experience that we live through, especially when repeated, enriches our Mirror System vocabulary most profoundly and in this way, by expanding our life experiences, we are increasingly able to understand the things we observe.

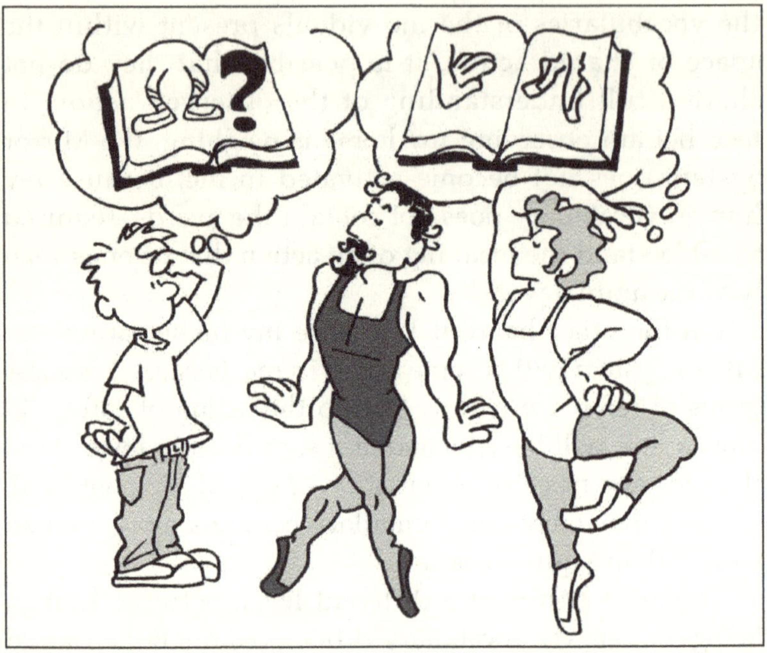

Fig. 15: vocabulary differences. When observing the ballet teacher, the boy's and the dancer's mirror system responses are different. While the mirror system is significantly activated in the dancer, given that he recognises a specific motor 'word' in each of the teacher's movements, in the boy this activation is quite weak, because he does not have the suitable motor 'words' that would enable him to fully appreciate his teacher's movements.

The role of emotions

What place do emotions occupy in relation to mirror neurons? Emotions add colour to our life and allow us to appreciate instantly the many aspects of the circumstances we find ourselves in, which is something that is necessary for both our survival and our social life. In fact, emotions affect our entire inner physiology (such as bowel movements, pain, pleasure, relaxation, contraction, etc.) and thus prime the entire body extremely quickly to be in the best possible shape to face up to whatever situation it finds itself in. How many times have you heard a sudden, loud noise and a shiver of fear has put you suddenly on the alert and ready for flight?

Of course this type of response may not always be appropriate as, for instance, when we are frightened for no reason. On the other hand, if emotions did not exist, we would not have the ability to respond to certain situations with the speed required to successfully escape from them. Emotions such as joy, pain, surprise, embarrassment, shame, sadness, anger, relief, satisfaction and so on play a crucial role, in that they give us the opportunity to quickly find our bearings in any context, particularly in social contexts.

So far we have looked at mirror neurons from a strictly motor-oriented viewpoint, as most related studies have actually been conducted in relation to the motor system. This is because it represents the most 'neutral' field of investigation for a clear and correct interpretation of the data. This does not mean that once the mechanism that underlies the motor Mirror System has been fully understood this awareness could not be transferred to other parts of our brain, such as those that govern emotions. Research studies have actually been conducted to ascertain whether humans have a Mirror System located in the areas reserved for emotions; to this end, the studies have focused on an area of the cerebral cortex called the *insula,* which processes feelings of pain and disgust and visceromotor integration, which consists of transforming sensory data into visceral reactions. Visceromotor integration is what allows emotions to have *colour,* and prevents them being reduced to some kind of cold cognitive perception.

Tests have been carried out to the effect that–whenever we observe a person who is experiencing either pain or

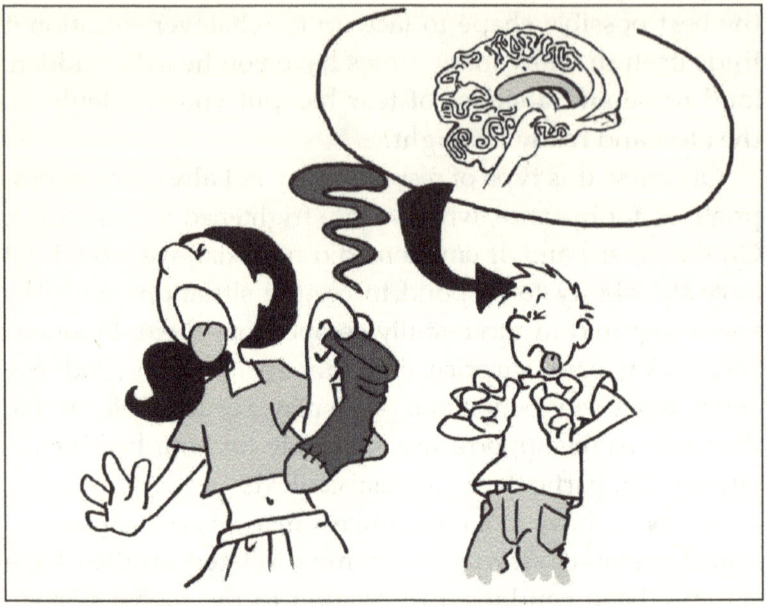

Fig. 16: activation of the insula. When observing a person who is experiencing a negative emotion such as pain or disgust, the same areas activated in the person who feels the pain or disgust, and which produce such state, is activated in our brain.

disgust–the same areas that are active in this person and which produce that state of pain or disgust are activated in us too, especially the insula (*Fig. 16*).

By observing others expressing their emotions, and by recognising the configuration of those expressions at motor level, the areas used to control emotions become immediately active, thus evoking in the observer a visceromotor response *similar to that of the person observed,* although such response does not possess the same intensity. Basically, we have the capacity *to enter into empathy* with the other person and to understand immediately his inner state, as this is actually reproduced within

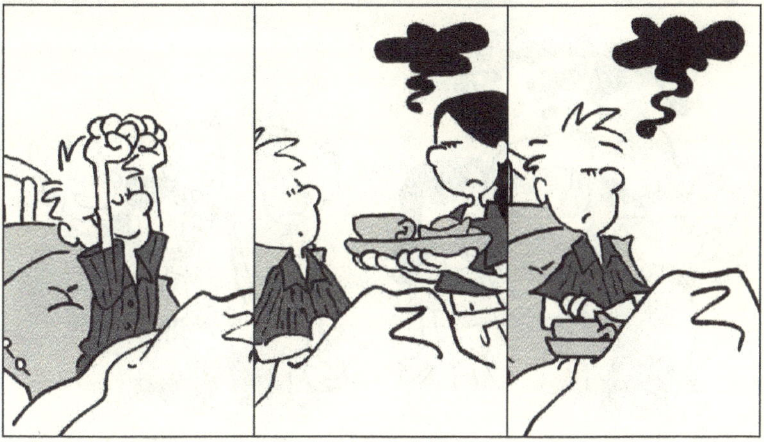

Fig. 17: shared empathic space. We immediately recognise others' emotions and we experience them ourselves, with an intensity that is directly proportional to the type of relationship we have with the other person.

ourselves. What is interesting to note, however, is that this response, although it *might be present* in us simply by observing the other person, can be significantly inhibited or facilitated depending on the type of role that the person fulfils for us. In the case of an enemy, the empathic intensity is drastically reduced, whereas in the case of a friend, it grows significantly, and one can reach the point of actually 'feeling' what the other feels. This demonstrates, even when it comes to emotions, the presence of a resonance mechanism that is similar to the motor Mirror System, and which enables us, every time we relate to others, to create a shared empathic space where others' emotions are evoked within us, in addition to being recognized and understood (*Fig. 17*).

As previously mentioned, this does not mean that we experience exactly what others do, because we must not forget that compassion (from the Greek 'suffering with'

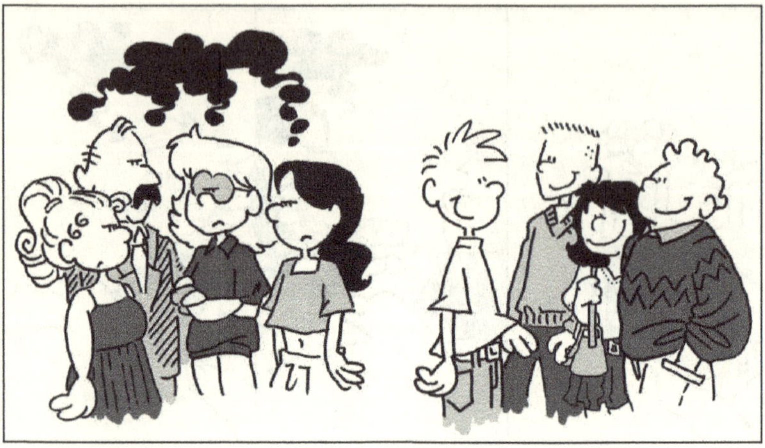

Fig. 18: shared empathic space. The emotions that we experience are shared amongst all those in our company or who simply observe us.

or 'feeling together') is strongly influenced by the type of role that the other fulfils in our eyes.

Imagine a situation in which we see someone crying: instantly we prepare ourselves to do the same, but we can also act in a different manner and hence not cry, but perhaps even laugh, depending on what the other person means to us and subject to the type of situation that has led the person to cry. The same equally applies to laughter, anger, and so on.

At any rate, the existence of a shared empathic space in which we are potentially *always* conscious of the emotions of others, on the basis that we automatically understand such emotions, brings us all closer together in a way that perhaps we had not even thought possible until now (*Fig. 18*).

Whether you are my enemy or my brother, I have the capacity to recognise pain in you and come into resonance with it by understanding and *experiencing it* myself, even if only for a short time.

Similarly, you are capable of recognising joy in me, and coming into resonance with it, by understanding and experiencing it yourself. This awareness allows us to reinterpret what the real meaning of social *responsibility* is for us.

CHAPTER 2

A daily discovery

Let's talk about us

Man is an extraordinary animal, equipped with exceptional tools that make him (always assuming he does not become extinct...) the dominant species on the planet, capable of decisively influencing the whole environment, both positively and negatively: which is why he is largely responsible for what happens. Humans are intelligent, they can communicate enormous amounts of information and opinions of varying degrees of complexity, as well as instructions of every type. We know that to accomplish all this, in addition to words, they also and especially communicate through their behaviour[18].

Many books and research studies have demonstrated the substantial difference between *what* is said and *how* it is said. It is a well-known fact that *non-verbal* communication is more important than the words that are uttered, given that the most important aspects of communication, perhaps even the most sincere ones, are inferred from attitude and demeanour. Consider silence, for instance: it is an

18 Desmond Morris, *Manwatching: A Field Guide to Human Behaviour*, Triad/Panther Books, 1977.

extraordinary tool, which can communicate much more than we usually think. Would you like some examples? Just imagine expressions like 'I love you', 'I care about you', 'I am happy to be with you', 'it is lovely to see you', 'at last we meet again': they all belong to the social and emotional sphere, and language makes them *substantially* different. Now try to imagine that you are communicating these phrases to a person within their appropriate contextual reference, and that you are doing it solely with your face, concentrating in particular on your eyes and mouth and without uttering a single word. We know very well that we can manage it quite successfully: everybody is capable of communicating these phrases simply by using facial expressions, either instinctively or after some basic practical training, unless they suffer from some objective physiological, motor, expressive or cognitive condition. A particular smile that comes with a certain expression in the eyes is enough to convey a limitless amount of positive messages, even in silence. By stating all this we simply wish to highlight a concept that has already been widely demonstrated in a number of studies as far back as 1939 by the UCLA professor Albert Mehrabian: namely that we communicate much more at a non-verbal level than through words and the way we say them.

We have already seen how our brain is equipped with the extraordinary ability to recognise the precise intended function or purpose of a particular action that we have observed. It is therefore easy to understand how most of the information that is contained in a message can actually be conveyed by non-verbal language, which possesses a faster data acquisition speed than any verbally communicated type of information. On the whole gestures, attitudes and behaviour tend to reach their destination much more rapidly than words. And what do they reach? Departing directly from the eyes, they end up reaching the mirror neurons.

What kind of face are you pulling?

Humans are equipped with an extremely high number of facial muscles, much higher than any other animal, due to their need to communicate on a constant basis and in a manner that is constantly evolving. This leads us to consider the logic that underpins the gestures that humans habitually perform, depending on the social context to which they belong. In effect, some gestures displayed by some African populations cannot be 'decoded' by individuals who have grown up in other parts of the world, where other cultures are predominant. Just think that some Asian cultures teach how to portray expressions that 'do not reveal' what the person is actually thinking (can they really do that?), with the specific intent of 'containing' one's emotions. In Western cultures there are currents of thought, particularly geared towards sales-oriented communication techniques, where they teach you to adopt a certain 'mask' in order not to allow emotions to be shown (just think about those fixed smiles), with equally debatable results (*Fig. 19*).

In our evolutionary and educational process it is evident that the social context in which we are brought up is aimed at creating a codification 'network' of gestural messages. The 'OK' gesture, for instance, which brings thumb and forefinger together, may be a positive message in one culture and a negative, even vulgar, one in others. The culture to which we belong leads us to develop a code of conventional gestures that we use daily within the society in which we live.

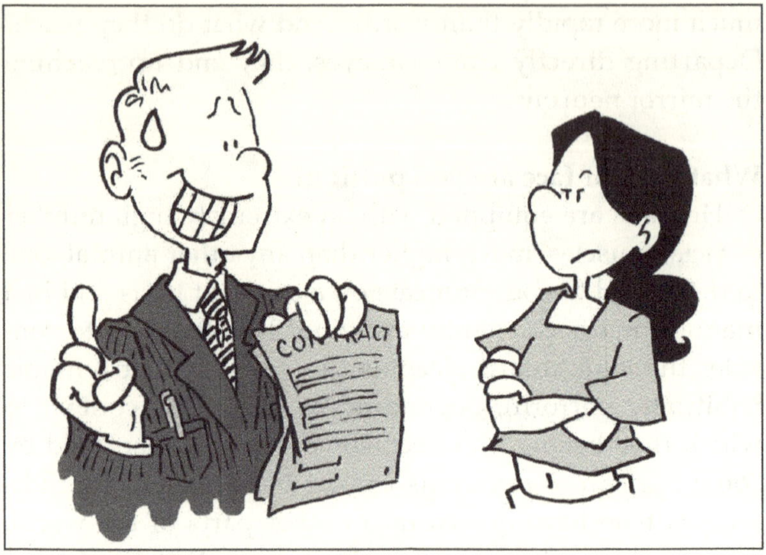

Fig. 19: does this salesperson inspire trust?

Every day we have the opportunity to observe countless common gestures that can be interpreted in a whole host of ways, ranging from handshaking (there is a proper and a not so proper way of doing it!) to kissing someone one has not seen for a long time on the cheek (be careful not to kiss them too passionately!), from talking to an acquaintance with a particularly loud voice (annoying, isn't it?) to countless different ways of walking (some are quite peculiar, don't you think?)

We have always imitated each other

Every day we are exposed to a huge number of signals, which we tend by and large not to notice or not to take into account simply because we either do not consider them relevant or because we have not developed the habit of noticing them. They are nonetheless an inexhaustible source of information, all geared towards our Mirror System, assuming they represent actions and gestures that we are familiar with.

You may think that this is like reinventing the wheel: well, essentially it is, however until now those deeper mechanisms that link our daily life with the mirror neuron system have been ignored. Most of all, behaviour that is functional to our goals and that exploits the Mirror System has not been widespread, at least not consciously.

Before we start considering the potential practical applications that stem from being aware of these mirror neurons, it is appropriate to take a few moments to reflect upon some questions. It is thought that humans are the most talented beings in the world when it comes to imitating one another. Take children for instance: when learning how to do any kind of action children are constantly focused on imitating others; they take their parents as models, or anyone who approaches them either by gesticulating or talking to them, and they attempt to imitate anything they see, hear or perceive in exactly the same way. When a child sees another child cry, it is highly likely that he or she will start crying too, and if he sees an adult smile, he is equally likely to smile in turn. How many mothers are, at this very moment, leaning over a cradle trying to teach their baby how to say 'mummy'? And how do they manage to teach this? They simply face the baby directly and slowly pronounce the word, repeating it tirelessly until one day that very word will escape from their child's lips. This is the same for virtually all motor-related learning, ranging from waving to eating, walking, up to and including performing countless daily activities. In the first months of life everything is taught by means of imitation. When language makes an appearance, there is an attempt to replace this imitation mechanism with an education *process* that revolves around 'issuing instructions' and which causes the growing child to put aside his extraordinary ability to imitate in order to make way for virtually unconscious actions. Just think if instead humans could become newly aware of their innate instinct to imitate: they would probably realise how many times they keep imitating even in adulthood, and without even realising it.

As they grow older, humans tend to forget that they possess this incredible capacity to learn from others through imitation and replace it with learning through words, words that, as shown by many studies on communication, seem to count for very little[19]. One of the aims of this book is to make us aware that this imitation mechanism that characterises human social relations does not become obsolete after the first few years of life but remains present as a latent capacity, which is taken for granted and neither practised nor valued as it should be.

The opportunities that would be unleashed from the conscious utilisation of this imitating ability, if turned into something just as powerful in adulthood, would be phenomenal.

Why did Leonardo da Vinci–like the majority of the extraordinary artists history has graced us with–teach students how to draw by allowing a few fortunate ones to observe him, in absolute silence, rather than sitting behind a desk and explaining it to them in theoretical

19 According to a 1967 study by the above-mentioned Albert Mehrabian, the importance of words amounts to 7%, compared to paraverbal (38%) and non-verbal communication (55%).

terms? The observation and imitation of others is the most powerful tool at our disposal for turning a huge amount of experience into something that is ours, which we can then easily transform into personal knowledge, thanks to both our cognitive abilities and outside information.

After all, how many times have we heard the expression 'watch and learn'?

We watch, and then we try

At this stage we could say that imitation is an everyday human mechanism that is perpetrated either consciously or unconsciously and that has enormous consequences. We have all noticed that if we see someone yawn, we are all seized by an unconscious urge to yawn and often do! Similarly, when we come across an acquaintance who is in a particularly sombre mood, we tend to *align ourselves* with that state (remember the famous resonance?), imitating it or at any rate *priming or predisposing ourselves* to experience it. And that is the key word: *predisposition.*

Whenever we observe someone carrying out an action, we predispose ourselves to repeat what we are observing, just as when we see someone experience an emotion, we predispose ourselves to relive it; this is why, when we are really gripped by a film and there is a tear-jerking scene we may well shed a little tear. And even if we do not, there is no doubt that at that moment our emotional state is decidedly more pronounced than before. This is why whenever we watch a gripping thriller we tend to jump at each dramatic turn of events (even our heartbeat and breathing seem to increase and our facial expressions change!), while we are nonetheless perfectly aware that it is nothing but pure fiction, and that very often we are only looking at computer-generated images and that the blood is not real but, as our grandparents used to say, just 'tomato sauce'!

We don't care if it is tomato sauce, or anything else for that matter, because it nevertheless evokes certain feelings in us, which often are not of a positive kind.

This automatic and uncontrollable mechanism is linked to the presence in our brain of the mirror neurons, another reason why it would be extremely useful if everyone was aware of the extraordinary consequences of this discovery: it is destined to change not only the way we all communicate, but also how we all live. A dear friend was telling us how as a little boy he would wait for his father to come home for dinner, and that before doing anything, he would wait and observe his father's expression once he had stepped through the front door. If his father opened the door with a relaxed expression on his face, he would run to him; and conversely, if he came in looking *stressed* or *angry*, he would wait before approaching him. This totally natural mechanism is based on the fact that the child initially observes his father and immediately perceives his mood, then *predisposes himself* to experience it, after which he decodes the mood *without any reasoning*, and only afterwards he reaches a decision on what to do. It is therefore clear that whatever action the little boy takes, it will inevitably be conditioned by the initial image of both his father's face and his attitude upon coming home.

Now that we have managed to clarify the imitation mechanism that humans experience unconsciously on a daily basis, let us return to the word *predisposition*. The action of seeing others experience a particular feeling will predispose us to experience it as well. Not everyone will be scared when watching a horror movie, some will remain perfectly indifferent, probably because they make a *rational* decision to remember that it is just fiction, or perhaps because their life experiences have caused them not to be frightened by certain images, or perhaps even because they might not be paying *much* attention to it.

Those who instead tend to observe what is being projected in a *participatory way* will consciously predispose themselves to experience the very feelings that the film is supposed to conjure up, and will for instance react with *fear* to those sequences that are aimed at generating that kind of reaction. Apart from anything else, this is exactly why the film was made in the first place!

There are many case studies regarding this predisposition. Think of a time when you were introduced to someone *new*: the moment of the introduction is extraordinary, because your mind is very busy decoding countless bits of information. If on that specific occasion your new friend was unfortunately suffering from a painful physical condition, his attitude might have seemed a bit *odd*, so much so that you might react by thinking that he himself might be a bit *odd* (*Fig. 20*). Without necessarily wanting to imitate his physical condition (a condition that you might not have been able to define as yet), you would certainly imitate his or her sense of discomfort, at least for a few moments, long enough to realise whether it is a real form of discomfort or something else. This quick transition towards a predisposition to discomfort will enable you to interpret and understand *what is odd*, and you will start this relationship in an *odd* manner. If however, to give a different example, you are introduced to a person who displays a good-humoured attitude right from the start, this will predispose you to approach him or her in a good-humoured manner. And so it goes, in that the effect of a relationship that begins in an *incongruous* way will

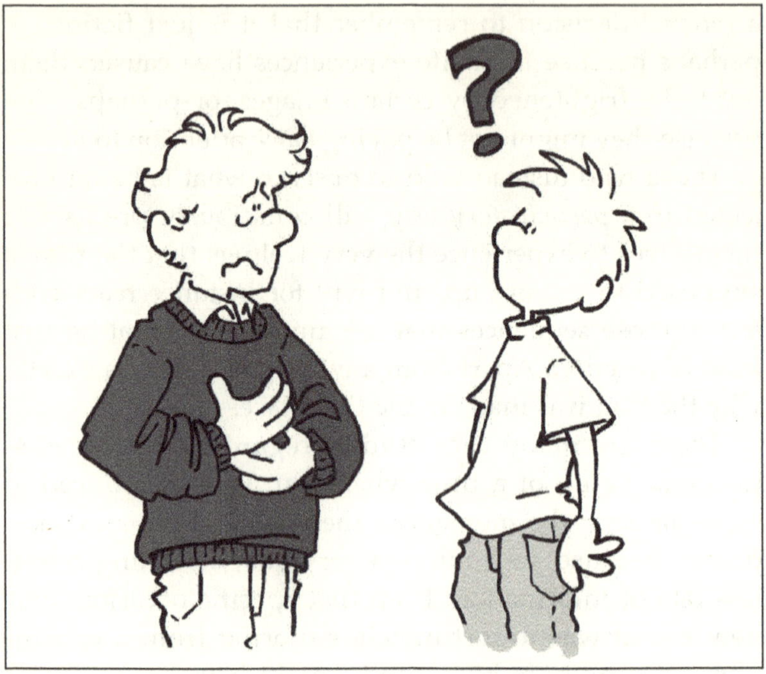

Fig. 20: let's imagine that we have been introduced to this person: clearly the first impression might not be great, in that his state of discomfort (the causes of which are unknown to us) will inevitably be communicated to us and will in turn cause us some discomfort.

most probably trigger off an equally incongruous continuation of that same relationship (something that we will go into in greater depth at a later stage in this book).

This also happens at the start of a work meeting or when we are about to begin collaborating with somebody. Just think what would happen if you were to show up at a meeting with your boss pulling a long face as a consequence of an earlier argument with your son, or if you were trying to make a sale while in the grip of a panic attack: all these details would immediately be noticed by others.

Some of you might have experienced going into a shop only to come across some particularly off-putting sales assistants. Just consider for a moment what effect their bad mood had on you at the beginning of your encounter: surely that put you in a bad mood too, froze the smile on your face and *prepared you for a potential clash.*

More specifically, what were their faces and expressions like when you walked into the shop? Did the fact that they welcomed you with this attitude trigger some specific reaction in you? And again: did their expressions, in your opinion, condition the outcome of the sale? These are all questions that suggest a number of obvious answers and these days they represent the main topic of many sales training courses.

Social responsibility

Using these sales techniques as a starting point, let us revisit the concept of social responsibility with the help of some examples that we will use throughout this chapter.

'Always smile', 'be courteous', 'answer and deal with people in a polite manner' are some of the rules that have guided our sales culture for a very long time and continue to do so. To this day, some training courses insist that trainees smile continuously. Why do we do this? We do it because mirror neurons show us that 'smiling is contagious' and therefore, if you really wish to make others smile, you must smile too! It sounds rather odd when put this way, because the very fact of *having to* smile may cause some people to ask themselves a few questions (such as, "and what if I don't have any reason to smile?"). Indeed, if we have not followed a careful motivational path beforehand, the outcome could well turn out to be that notorious *fake smile,* which possesses one extraordinary feature: it can be spotted, identified and classified almost immediately! And why is that, we may wonder? Now we know the answer.

In some way we are actually responsible for other people's emotions. If we are sad, we will sadden those who see us and this, *if we are aware of it, can be avoided.*

Until now it seemed that mirror neurons were a topic exclusively for scientists, for those who analysed the subject from a scientific standpoint; and yet, these *friends* of ours are a constant presence in our lives. Understanding the marvellous usefulness of the *mirrors* is indeed easier than we think, and this gives everyone some extraordinary opportunities to improve themselves.

Consider children again: these little men or women hide certain abilities that 'grown-ups' do not even dare imagine, starting with their amazing 'imaginary' fantasy skills. Children project hallucinations virtually everywhere, especially when they decide to play and they do not happen to have the object of their game to hand: they imagine that a shrub is a fabulous castle, or they arm themselves with cardboard swords and armour, not to mention their ability to concoct juicy dishes out of pebbles, twigs and grass. Children project images and, when they 'see' these images, they experience feelings.

Similar to this phenomenon typical of childhood is what in adulthood is often colloquially referred to as 'making your own movie', whereby we use our imaginations in quite a wasteful and useless manner. Are these movies always of a positive nature? Often they are not. More often than not the images that we show ourselves are not totally 'beneficial'. It is enough to imagine a negative work situation to make us sad, or to recall an unpleasant event that may have occurred years ago.

Tapping into those abilities that are typical of our imagination, we are extremely skilled at conditioning ourselves by projecting and 'hallucinating' unfavourable scenarios, painful possibilities, or even catastrophic consequences for our possible choices in life. Fair enough, in the sense that we are all free to imagine any images we want, all potential scenarios, including those catastrophic ones that are available to our imagination (although we might wonder why we are so keen to generate negative, rather than positive projections). What we really want to emphasise in this respect is that everything that we project, everything that we imagine, the castles, heavens or hells that we manage to create with our imagination, powerfully condition our emotions.

The really interesting aspect that once again draws attention to our social responsibility is that by conditioning ourselves so negatively we also change the mood and perceptions of all who come into contact with us and who are predisposing themselves to automatically imitate us. And, as we can guess, this is far from kind. We are therefore talking about something *hygienic*: we all know that giving off a bad smell is not hygienic and it is inappropriate towards everyone around us. Similarly, giving vent to a negative emotion, possibly created by our own imagination, is equally inappropriate, although located on a different plane from the sense of smell: just as in the case of a bad smell, a negative emotion can afflict others too!

If anything, this process is an unconscious one, and therefore now that we are aware of its existence, we can decide to make different choices, producing undoubtedly better results.

With a little bit of training we could, for instance, still encounter failure and yet make a conscious decision to focus on the positive lesson that it brings, thus projecting a happy and lucky scenario, and experiencing positive (and 'contagious') feelings. On the other hand, we could decide to ruin what is potentially a peaceful life by wasting our time in thinking about some hypothetical misfortunes that could befall us or our loved ones, whose likely outcome would be some deeply negative (and equally 'contagious') emotions.

This kind of power, which lies in our hands, is actually a result of the fact that these flights of fancy are actually totally *visible* to everyone. Yes, it is true: when we feel sad, it is noticeable and when we are happy, it is equally noticeable. It all seems so obvious and yet we ought to give more consideration to the fact that, even when we pretend to be happy, it is quite noticeable that we are just pretending!

We have a wide selection of scripts at our disposal that we may decide to recite in our daily acting, but although we may well be wonderful actors, other people's mirror neurons will be able to detect such minute nuances that deceiving them will be nigh impossible. People who observe us are capable of perceiving infinitely subtle aspects of our emotions, sometimes even the ones that are most definitely hidden.

Are you still convinced that it is worth spending even a single minute projecting some future unfavourable scenario for yourselves? Or might it not be more interesting *to build* positive effects to juxtapose with our future actions and attitudes? If nothing else, those close to us would thank us for it, just as we ourselves feel more at ease when we happen to interact with balanced people. A peaceful and positive emotion is much more willingly imitated, as we are naturally drawn to it!

Certainly, going into a job interview thinking: "I will never get the job" has an inversely proportional effect on one's recruitment chances, as it conditions even the most imperceptible micro-movements of both body and face, and gives the interviewer some very precise information as regards one's confidence and motivation, among other things. The same holds true in relation to sitting a school exam thinking beforehand: "I will never pass". The first person to notice such 'omens' of ours (and perhaps even become convinced of them) will be the teacher, having perfectly deciphered our mood and emotions.

In the following chapters we will deal with these and other practical aspects.

CHAPTER 3

Observation: an instrument for action

We improve through observation

In the previous chapter we gave numerous examples in an attempt to prove one particular fact: observing others in an active and attentive manner enables us to detect much more than we would otherwise gather from simple, passive listening and observation.

However, what is the point of such careful observations? Let's cast our minds back to all those situations in which we asked ourselves: "What can I improve about myself?" To this deceptively simple question we have often given answers that have led to actions aimed at reaching certain specific goals.

If, for instance, we were wondering about how to improve our communication skills, one way of achieving such a laudable aim might have been to read one or two books or perhaps take a training course. Such courses or books clearly revolve around how to communicate more effectively, how to manage interpersonal relationships, or how to resolve conflicts: there is no shortage of relevant books and training courses on offer. But what are the contents that really interest us? These products often focus on *what to do, how to do it, what attitude, and what actions* to take in order to achieve better performances in line with our objectives. The question that we can ask ourselves at this stage is: do these tools *definitely* work? And are they effective with *every type* of audience? Does speaking in public have fixed rules or does it depend on the audience? Does managing a successful relationship with one's friends, partners or colleagues entail fixed rules? The spontaneous reply to these simple questions is easy to guess, and it is a 'no'. What to do then? First of all it is certainly advisable to have a 'toolbox' equipped with such literary or scientific products at your disposal and to make it your own. After which, it could be useful to integrate these techniques with the wonderful tool of observation.

Active observation, the queen amongst mankind's instruments of knowledge, enables us both to be flexible and adaptable, and through observation we can continuously appreciate all those aspects and nuances that turn a specific circumstance into something unique.

This is where mirror neurons come into play. It is actually the ability of our Mirror System to understand in real time the very essence of what others are doing and experiencing that allows us to develop a full understanding of communicative relationships, in that it provides our observation with the indispensable speed required to come up with suitable and *appropriate* answers to circumstances, well beyond any rigid patterns.

We attend training courses or simply read books and study their suggestions in order to better handle certain activities such as speaking in public, or managing conflicts, or even just communicating effectively. There are many excellent tools available that we can call upon: what is crucial to point out is that the circumstances to which these techniques are applied will never be identical. Even

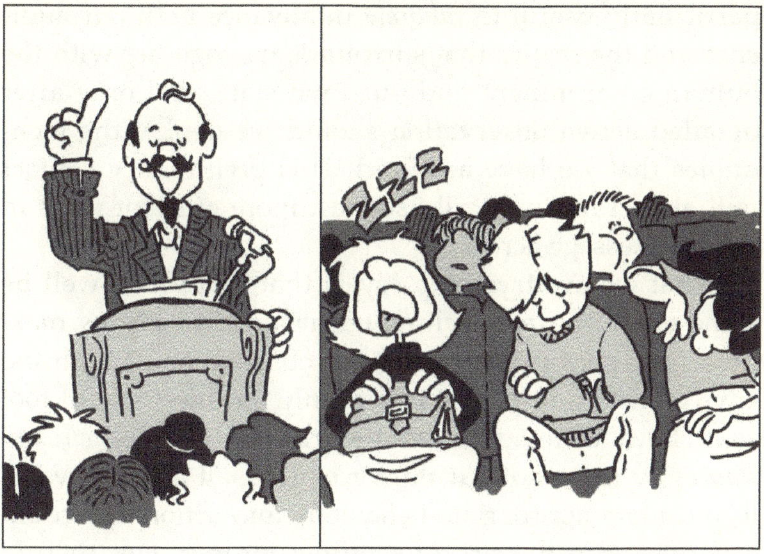

Fig. 21: clearly this speaker does not possess a well-developed mirror system, given that he has not realised that he has completely lost the attention of his audience.

the same audience in exactly the same location, after one hour has elapsed, will have changed: the context is in constant evolution and with every new evolution, new observations become necessary. These changes do make a difference, together with the perception that we have of them, and the mood that both we and the people that we relate to are in. For this reason we need a tool that enables us to quickly read and assess the circumstances: this *gift* is embodied in our Mirror System. Active observation is one way to make the best use of our Mirror System and it gives us the ability *to adjust ourselves,* i.e. to adapt ourselves to the circumstances (*Fig. 21*).

Let's proceed further and, rather than taking our own message into consideration, it will be equally and particularly useful to *calibrate* in advance both our audience and the reality that surrounds us, together with the human environment and our own state, and only after detailed active observation should we deploy the techniques that we have acquired. This preliminary contact will almost automatically suggest more efficient ways to get our message across.

What we are trying to say is that there may well be some extraordinary techniques around to help us maximise our performances, but the observation of both the environment and people is certainly our most useful tool as it allows us to appreciate the *true reality of these circumstances* by means of our mirror neurons. It also allows us to put more appropriate behaviour into action. We could otherwise run the risk of sending out messages that do not serve our purpose to a person or a group of people who have no interest in our message, resulting in ineffective communication on our part.

Observing and acting

It may seem unbelievable, but observation and action do not always follow in that order. People often act first, *then* observe the outcome of their actions. It looks like a strategic error, does it not? Just think about all those occasions when we have said something, only to regret it afterwards, ("I should have bitten my tongue!"), or when we do something rash that gives rise to unforeseen results and are left to observe its unwanted effects. Could these consequences have been avoided? The answer to this question belongs to the field of philosophical logic, yet we would like to invite our readers to reflect on a 'change of strategy', on a U-turn from a time standpoint: what would happen if we were to observe first and then act?

Observation is targeted at our mirror neurons and allows us to come into resonance with others, providing us with extremely important information. It enables us to understand the predisposition of those in front of us, their degree of attentiveness, their willingness to listen to us, their emotional state and so on.

Afterwards, thanks to our *internalising* all these implied messages sent by our audience, which have reached us through the mirror neurons, we can act and communicate our message more effectively. At this juncture our communication will take into account all the micro-messages, especially the non-verbal ones, the listener himself (or the group) has sent us. Even a simple blink of the eyes, a frown, a smile or a scowl can be very useful signals for understanding the environment (in the sense of both human and spatial environment) in which we find ourselves.

Those of us who before communicating anything to anyone have decided to try to actively observe the other party's non-verbal signals (face, features, countenance, breathing, posture, in other words absolutely everything!), easily realise that the message we then communicate will be vastly more effective than when we do not observe. This is because our *mirrors* rapidly come up with a suggestion as to the other person's *state,* which once encoded allows our cognitive abilities to decide how to act accordingly. Just try and see for yourselves.

We recommend a reasonable level of patience and some good training in observation skills.

To recap, whenever we interact with anyone, if *before* acting we were to observe the state of the people with whom we have decided to connect, and were to *listen* to the data coming from our Mirror System, our ensuing message would be much more effective, as it would be

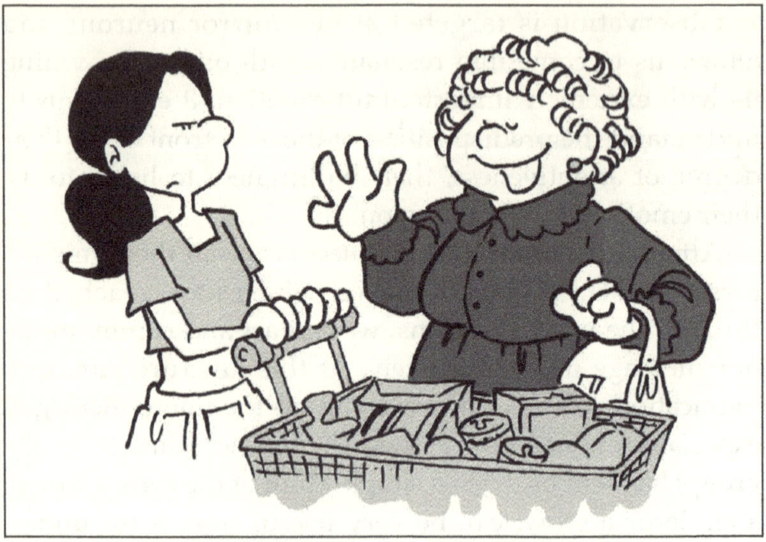

Fig. 22: the elder woman is not paying any attention to her own emotional mirror system, otherwise she might have realised by now that the young woman does not appreciate her action.

'appropriate' to the signals issued by the person in front of us. Needless to say, before any of this we should carefully check what message *we* are sending others (and not just verbally!), and then check our own emotions, because this is an element that will very definitely produce a conditioning effect on others.

Here is a simple example: have you ever been in a hurry to run an important errand, only to come across someone who greets you warmly and then embarks upon an account of his or her day in detail? It is quite annoying and yet that person is not even remotely aware that you are in a rush, nor of your total unwillingness to listen (*Fig.* 22). If only he or she had the patience to observe you before they opened their mouth, they would realise that 'now is not the time'. How much would our relationships change if everyone were to pay more attention to these messages communicated directly by the mirror neurons?

Innate imitation

Our sight is responsible for that extraordinary process that we have already discussed, namely imitation. As we have already said, children grow up imitating and when an adult decides to imitate the gestures of a child, in the eyes of the child he or she will certainly appear much nicer than those adults who busy themselves with 'grown up' activities. Children simply love observing adults who behave like them. Try it. Through our sight we process countless amounts of information, which we link to actions, feelings, emotions, memories and so on. The simple observation of an image is sufficient for our brain to activate a series of neural areas, depending on the memory and the feeling that we have linked to the sight of the actual image. Sometimes it is also sufficient for us to look at somebody to even understand his or her most profound motivation, or the emotional state they are in. After all, and as widely demonstrated, it is those non-verbal aspects of communication that can reveal the emotions that go beyond words: attitudes, gestures, expressions, at times even a person's charisma, are all indications that are perceived by us through sight, and it is our Mirror System, in conjunction with what emerges from visual signals, that is giving us most of this information. A charismatic person will succeed in attracting the attention of others spontaneously and will do so as soon as others see him or her and spot his or her charismatic 'aura'. There is nothing particularly esoteric about this: it is simply that, *instinctively,* once we have seen a particular person, we often have a sense of whether or not we can trust him or her. Just as it is possible to utter the sentence: "something tells me that he is deceiving me", even though we may not have necessarily 'heard any rumours' alerting us to any potential deception by someone, but have simply looked at somebody and perceived their unreliability. But what is it that makes this person *look* unreliable? Probably the fact that he or she is acting in a manner that is not in tune with the moral principles that they purport to follow, or which they know they ought to abide by, is inexorably *expressed* by some micro-movement of the face or body, which directly reaches our friends the mirror neurons and enables us to *encode* the 'I do not trust him'.

Think of when you do something you are not sure you want to do: do you do it in a relaxed or in a rigid way? It is easy to tell when a smile is false, just as we often spot when some smart aleck is trying to take us for a ride, or is simply saying something not quite true (and knows it full well).

On the other hand–to return to the example of the charismatic individual–a person who is balanced and in tune with his or her principles and values, convinced of what he or she is doing, will behave in an appropriate manner. We see this and immediately translate it into: "I trust him". The steps are: I observe, I feel and I decide. In this case, we have observed a balanced person, we have felt this balance within us by coming into resonance with him through the Mirror System and finally we have translated all this into a "we can trust him". Conversely, in the case of an incongruous person, we would have similarly observed, felt a sense of incongruence or unease, and translated all this into: "I do not trust him".

We are making a very important statement here: in our daily actions it is crucial that before acting we stop for a moment to check the congruence of our actions with our objectives, wishes and values; basically to understand if we really want to carry out a particular action, because if we do not, it will be clear that we do not want to do it. This is because doing something that we are not keen on makes us incongruous and that is easily recognisable!

Clearly we cannot like everything that we have to do. What matters is to be aware that others will realise perfectly well that we do not like it, as inevitably they can discern our emotions, thanks to their Mirror System.

Observation makes us "feel" some amazing things. Long before anyone knew about mirror neurons Adam Smith[20] was able to say something as amazing as this: "When we see that a blow is about to be dealt to someone's leg or arm, we instinctively step back and pull our own leg or arm back; and when the blow actually lands, somehow we feel it too and suffer from it just like the victim."

Amazing, isn't it? Such a precise description that accurately explains the type of mechanism that we experience on a daily basis: first we see and then we feel (internally). Sentences like: "I know how you're feeling", "I know what you're thinking" and "I can see how you are" are excellent examples of how visible our emotions are to everybody.

Talking of quotations, Charles Darwin himself gave us the following testimony: "If, when performing in public, a singer's voice turns a bit hoarse, many of the people in the room, as I have been assured by someone I trust implicitly, start coughing to clear their own throats [...] I have also been told that during a sport competition, when an athlete jumps up, many spectators [...] shuffle their feet".

Mutual imitation is clearly an innate human instinct.

20 An 18th-century Scottish philosopher and economist.

Acting appropriately

We often act according to what we have seen and felt and this plays to our advantage, as we can decide what part of ourselves we would like "to reveal". If we decide to go out on a day when we feel particularly negative, it might be useful to call upon our self-awareness and "rearrange" our emotions, first of all so that we feel better, but equally because if we don't, we would be sending others a huge number of negative signals, which would inevitably be translated (and possibly even copied).

Would you like an example? Would you like people to think that you are feeling sad? Or perhaps depressed? Would you appreciate it if they viewed you as someone negative? It is obvious that all these emotions can be detected very easily in others, but this incredible ease equally enables others to detect it just as easily in us! This is why it is advisable to observe our emotions first and figure out whether they are congruent with what we are about to do and only then act: this way the attitude that other people will be able to observe in us will be "cleaner" and they will have a more positive idea of us, which will improve our relationship.

We could call it *emotional contagion* simply on the basis that people tend to imitate others' manifestations of happiness, joy, anxiety, pain, disgust, as well as anything that can be expressed through mimicry and gestures. Other people accurately pinpoint these messages and tend to imitate them. We all know about the well-known yawning contagion, but it is now equally clear to us that smiling, joy, tenderness and fun are contagious too and don't you think that these are decidedly more "interesting"?

If we think about it, the lack of awareness of this imitating mechanism often leads us to paradoxical situations. For example, imagine a teacher who, driven to distraction by a noisy class, bursts out: "Shut up! That's enough! Enough!" (*Fig. 23*). It is conventionally thought that a human being at the receiving end of a stimulus would interpret it by following some complex processes and only later produce a response. In reality, however, human beings *experience* the stimulus produced by what they see or feel immediately through the functioning of their mirror neurons. The response can arrive virtually instantaneously, which is why the teacher who overreacts by shouting 'opens the neuronal doors' of his students to the specific action of 'shouting'. The effect of his "Shut up!" will probably not lead to silence, but will infect the classroom with the same mood as the teacher: anger, for instance, so that the class continues to make a noise, but with an added predisposition towards anger: totally the opposite outcome to the teacher's original intentions.

Although the teacher may be trying to do his duty and calm the class down, what he *does not know* is that by acting this way he is having the opposite of the desired effect, whereas it would be better if he were to endeavour to attain a 'calmer' state.

Or we can perhaps imagine a mother who anxiously tells her daughter, when gripped by a panic attack: "Calm down, calm down!" She cannot hope but produce a rise in anxiety!

All this has an even wider scope: just think about all those teenagers who are struggling with the latest generation of videogames. We are all aware that some extremely violent videogames are available on the market, where players can perform unbelievably brutal actions at the expense of other humans. Sadly it has been established that the mere visual exposure to these scenarios can

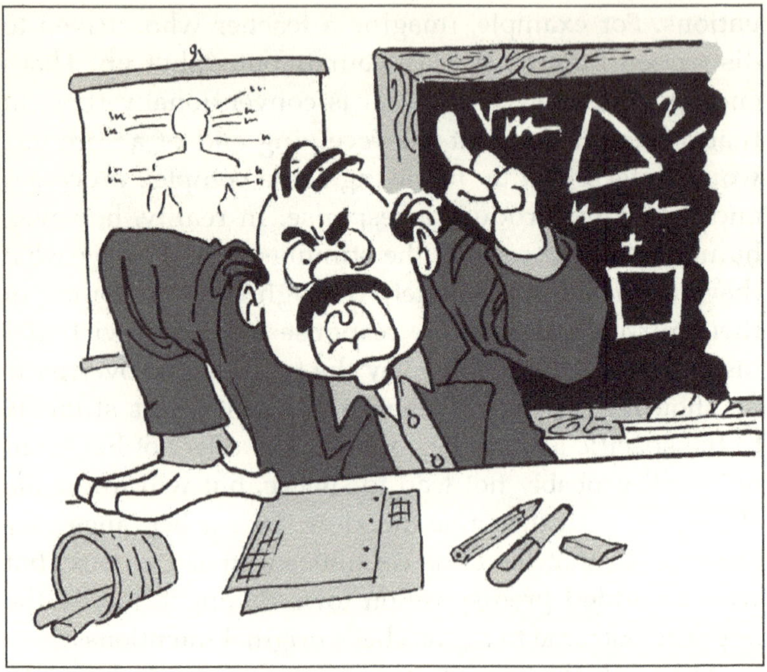

Fig. 23: a teacher like this one, who is trying to restore silence in the classroom by shouting like a madman, will probably not achieve great results!

trigger off some very violent behavioural patterns. The University of Huddersfield in the UK has recently shown how children become more aggressive after spending an afternoon playing a game of virtual football. Back in 2000, the *Journal of Personality and Social Psychology* published an article in which it was claimed that, in addition to increased aggression, some videogames might be responsible for poorer school results. According to its two researchers, namely Craig A. Anderson of the University of Missouri and Karen E. Dill of Rhyne College, the effects of violent videogames linger on over time in individuals who have been negatively impacted by them.

"Even a brief exposure to some violent videogames", the two scientists write, "can temporarily accelerate an aggressive type of behaviour."

This is tantamount to saying that even if we were just to witness a violent action, we would become *a little more violent* in turn, or at least we would predispose ourselves to become so. Many research studies have shown that there is a clear correlation between exposure to the violence portrayed in the media and the build-up of violent behaviour over time. After all, if a romantic film can move us, a drama make us cry, and a horror movie scare us, what could be the effect on us of a violent film?

We are not yet used to managing these dynamics, although we are now aware of them but the time has thus come to take full possession of them and through this improve the interpersonal relationships in our everyday life.

Act within groups

Think of the empathy that develops at either a concert or a political rally. Groups act as great feeling amplifiers because inside a group everything is multiplied and the imitation mechanism is virtually instantaneous. Take the example of a football stadium, when strong empathy, or perhaps even downright panic, develop among the supporters. In concerts too, the emotions generated are "shared" in an extraordinary way. We have a tendency to observe ourselves and when we do it actively, we predispose ourselves to imitate other people's emotions, even when we simply watch them being portrayed on a cinema screen. Many of us will have experienced what we go through in the course of a sports event involving two opposite factions: the stadium literally splits into two, and being part of one of the two factions renders the individuals belonging to the same group homologous. This explains why when someone in the group starts to shout, they all begin to shout, and likewise if one of them were to laugh, they would all progressively be inclined towards laughter too. This is very helpful for understanding numerous phenomena of a social nature, such as panic: the type of panic that can develop in a stadium or in a crowded place can lead to tragedy simply because, when they see that a whole group of people is starting to run, everyone else will set off running too. In a concert it is wonderful to become collectively excited, but it is equally true that, owing to those same dynamics, when someone decides to turn violent in a "lively" demonstration, many others will probably be prepared to follow suit. The somewhat improvised yet effective water cannon used by police forces is specifically intended to "separate" the human block that has been formed. Groups can be extraordinary when they gather together for positive purposes, but they can be equally powerful–and dangerous, particularly to their own members–to negative ends.

To give a positive example, as the saying goes, there is *strength in numbers*, right? Nature teaches us some amazing things in this respect: just think about a shoal of tiny fish that when moving in perfect unison take on the appearance of one huge fish, hence managing to frighten off their predators (who fall for the trick, thinking that they are facing one massive fish). In this example all the fish imitate each other and in so doing create a compact mass. Mirror neurons are extraordinary when functioning within groups, and they manage to make even incredibly large masses move in unison. This same phenomenon can be witnessed even in smaller groups: just think about when we say that in a particular company: "they are all made from the same mould", or of people who do a particular job, "you can spot them a mile off ". It is interesting to discover that there is a significant element of truth in these expressions, due to the fact that when we join a group, we tend to conform to their behaviour and the way they speak and even, dare we say, the way they think.

Hello?

Now we would like to mention something that should not be overlooked, which is linked to what we "observe through our ears". Take telephone calls: how many times, just on the basis of the initial "Hello?" have you developed a rather accurate idea (or perhaps you have predisposed yourselves to create one) of the mood of the person that has answered your call? Well, often what happens is that after a particularly breathless "Hello?" we say, "I'm sorry, am I disturbing you? Shall I ring you back later?" This is really an assumption (created by the predisposition), yet it can be found in many practical examples, which each and every one of us has experienced directly at some point. We have assumed that the person that answered us was in a particularly unsuitable setting to talk to us and have therefore adapted ourselves to this feeling by acting accordingly and suggesting an alternative. We often hear the reply, "No problem at all", and at that stage our assumption instantaneously vanishes. Why did we have this wrong initial idea? Simply because our mirror neurons had detected a peculiar and perhaps unusual tone of voice in the person we rang and they had acted as if we had used that tone of voice. The ensuing process was therefore a sort of, "If I were him and I replied in such a breathless tone, that would undoubtedly be because it is not convenient at the moment." We try to act as a "mirror" even on the phone, and this happens very often. Think about the sentence: "What's the matter? You sound a bit funny..." which is repeated on the phone who knows how many times a day. Even a minute and seemingly imperceptible slur in either one's voice or breathing can be detected on the phone and encoded by the listener's mirror neurons.

Actually, it would often be quite useful to carry out a quick self-inspection of one's own emotional state before answering the phone, as it would save a lot of time that otherwise would be wasted in trying to clear up any misunderstandings.

The above example helps us reflect on how these mirror neurons are not only activated by sight, but also by hearing, and in an extremely fascinating way to boot. The only restriction lies in the fact that a simple acoustic signal carries less information when compared to a complete communicative relationship in which it is possible to observe the body as well. It is obvious, therefore, that if we can "see" the other person we are in much better contact with the reality of the events than when we just hear the voice.

Think about somebody who has the habit of talking while chewing or when they are lying down. We can then appreciate how many 'distortions' may occur in a telephone conversation, and how much information is conveyed by these distortions to our Mirror System in relation to the real or the assumed state of the other person (speaking lying down, or with a full mouth) and thus cause a number of misunderstandings at multiple levels. In the case of a work-related phone call first thing in the morning, for instance, we would usually expect to be at the receiving end of a clear and lively answer, as this type of correspondence has become crystallised in our mental associations. If, however, we receive a muffled reply and our Mirror System recognises, for instance, a tone of voice typically associated with someone who is lying down, a sense of incongruence is born in us, which is rapidly overcome the moment that we recognise that the other person has just woken up.

It is clear that when we also have access to visual observations we are in possession of much more information and this enables us to lessen the chances of any potential *misunderstandings.*

This is why in our opinion both sight and observation are fundamental for understanding others, above and beyond other communication channels.

CHAPTER 4

Congruence and emotions

Imitating sincerity

Let's go back to the *fake smile* that we came across in Chapter 1. When someone's smile is fake and insincere, we all tend to notice it and when it is displayed by people that we have known for some time, it is even more noticeable. Why is this? Once again, when we see someone smile in a particular way, thanks to the Mirror System a corresponding state is evoked within ourselves, which predisposes us to smile in a manner identical to that we have observed. As we have seen, all this takes place so quickly that we don't even realise it: this is due to the action of the Mirror System, through mechanisms that are filtered prior to reaching the reasoning phase and that evoke in us a state that corresponds to what is being observed (independently of our will). The only thing that we are likely to say is: "that is a fake smile". How have we inferred all this? Irrespective of how, all of you have experienced this, and in this sequence, hundreds of times.

At this juncture it is evident that 'telling lies' is not such a good idea, as it only requires someone who has established good contact with their own Mirror System through a modicum of observation to show us up. This contact, or ability to listen to one's own Mirror System, is what we are usually describing when we say: "You are so sensitive!"

Just think about the number of times we have been listening to somebody on the TV, only to realise instantly that they were not saying exactly what they were thinking. Or perhaps, as we listen to some friend's advice, we realise that they themselves do not sound really convinced and therefore we choose to follow our own counsel. The intention of the authors of this book is directed at those "professional liars", to whom we'd like to send our well-meaning message: be careful, because since people discovered the way mirror neurons work, you are going to be found out much more easily!

Congruence

The example of the fake smile introduced a new element that we had already defined as *incongruence*. To explain it in more detail, it originates the moment we carry out an action without conviction, or perhaps unwillingly, or when this action does not express in the slightest what we are actually feeling. Incongruence happens when our non-verbal behaviour is not aligned with the objective of the action that we are in the process of performing, or with the words that we are saying, in other words, when there is no correspondence between emotional state, motor activity and mental state in the fulfilment of a targeted action. Think of when we would really like to be convincing, and yet our hands and gestures betray our insecurity.

Congruence on the other hand is the actual *participation* in the action that is unfolding: practically any action is possible. Some specific examples: what distinguishes a good actor from a less gifted one? Consider two actors who are both skilled in the art and techniques of acting. "The difference is that on actor who communicates more and better", could be an answer, and it is effectively a correct answer, however it overlooks the fact that 'communicating more' depends on the emotional response generated by one of the two actors, as opposed to the other. If the actor acts in a totally congruent manner, that is to say 'enters' 100% into the character, then you could truly declare that person a great actor. If, however, the actor maintains a certain emotional coldness and does not enter into the role (unless portraying him or herself), then you will perceive a dystonia and incongruence, which we encode as: "I think I know what he is trying to get across, but he can't manage it at present". This is then be easily translated as "he does not communicate anything to me", or possibly "he is not a good actor".

Alternatively think about a time when you were criticised in a very hurtful way and endeavoured to hide the way you felt inside thinking it was a "weakness", showing instead a complete lack of emotions: unless we happen to be excellent actors, this leads us to manifest incongruence.

Congruence results from a harmony between our actions, our moods or emotions and our intentions. When these three factors are properly oriented towards what we wish to achieve, then the result will be a congruent action.

Knowing this helps us to throw some light onto a situation that is very widespread these days: the inability to recognise one's own *alignment with the role*. The role that we play, be it at work or within the framework of society, *demands* that we possess certain specific qualities–and not any others–that would allow us to attain the results that we are after in a fluid and unimpeded way. In performing our role it is highly desirable to possess the type of moti-

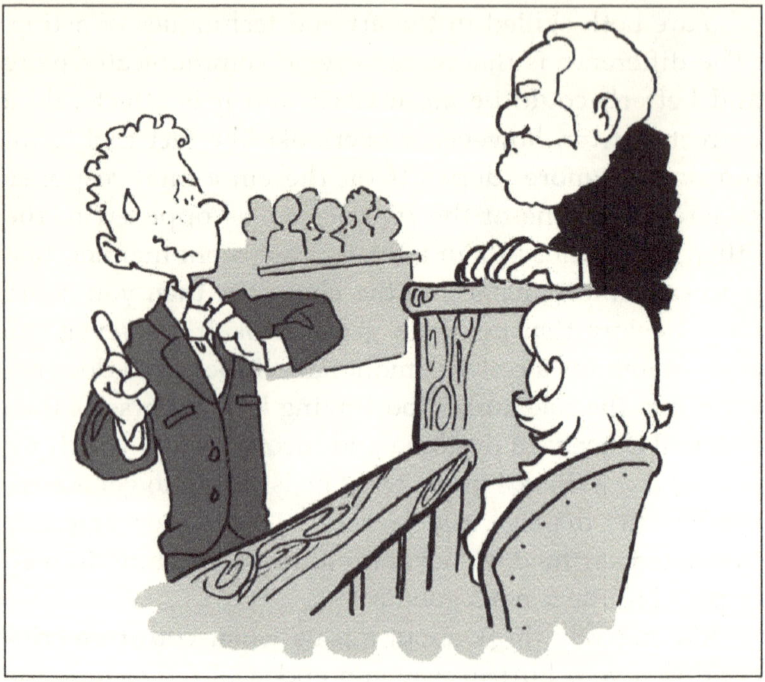

Fig. 24: this young lawyer is not well aligned with his role, as he is not paying attention to what he is communicating both through his gestures and through his expressions. In so doing he conveys insecurity, while he should appear confident and determined.

vation that will keep on spurring us to maintain a constant alignment with the role and remain congruent with its required manifestations.

We often come across people who however *do not wish* to play their role *in the slightest,* which translates into an inharmonious relationship between what they are supposed to be doing and their intentions (i.e. to do something completely different). Inevitably these people will appear visibly incongruous, namely in terms of their attitude, their way of speaking and so on.

Imagine a conversation with an employer: while we are talking about something important we notice that he is looking out of the window, fiddling with his pencil, looking at his watch, slouching and munching peanuts. Although he is there apparently listening to us, his attitude and behaviour are communicating anything but interest and attention on his part and we immediately perceive this as incongruence. There is effectively a major difference between his current mood and what he wants to or should communicate to us, i.e. his interest. As it clearly transpires, he *is not aligned* with his role, but he is unable to recognise it, as he is not paying attention to anything that he is communicating through his gestures, which are immediately decoded by our Mirror System (*Fig. 24*). This happens often and totally unwittingly, because he, like most of us, is not fully aware that every single movement of ours can be read by others like an open window into our inner state. Other people notice our incongruence virtually immediately and *they are aware of what we are doing.*

The discovery of mirror neurons will lead us to pay more attention to the level of congruence that we show in our communication, now that the external evidence of actions that are not aligned with our intentions has been demonstrated. So, if we do something without being mentally "aligned" with it, it is going to be noticed!

Nuances and strategies

How many times do we encounter people and ask them immediately how they are?

Very often their reply is: "Fine, thank you!" Yet when this happens, if we pay attention to their answers by carefully observing the other person, we will soon realise that of the many, "Fine, thank you!" replies that we receive some are congruent, while others are not.

It is quite straightforward to observe the countless variations within all these "Fine, thank you!" replies from movements, posture and facial expressions or, more simply, intuitively, which we could regard as the result of perceiving all those details that, although escaping our consciousness, fall nonetheless within the scope of our senses and come to be understood as they pass through our Mirror System. As we have seen already, this is even more evident whenever our observation decides to intervene to "give voice to our intuition", thus establishing a better contact with the Mirror System. When we compare what we observe in each of these answers, which on the level of language may well appear identical, we can then identify some "Fine, thank you!" replies that to us sound like, "Not at all fine!" or "Neither good nor bad, this is a habit-conditioned automatic reply". We are thus confronted with many examples of incongruence which, as we know, cannot escape our Mirror System, although they may easily not be picked up by cognitive processes alone.

A friend of ours who is involved in human resources management was involved in recruitment and was consequently involved with some young people looking for work. As he was reflecting on the qualities that might lead him to regard some candidates as "better" than others, in his attempt to interpret above all the needs of the company recruiting them, he could not help reaching a fundamental conclusion: the working world has changed and it is moving at an unpredictable speed. The professional skills required of workers years ago have changed radically and are in constant evolution: traditional technical skills are making way for new skills that are increasingly in demand; self-control, for instance, in the sense of the ability to recognise (and know how to manage) the emotions we display. Basically, if you are about to fly into a rage, you can become aware of it in advance (or during the process) and control this "temptation" and not give in to it.

Nothing revolutionary in that, if we think that even Aristotle in his *Nicomachean Ethics* stated that: "the problem does not reside in the emotion itself, rather in the *appropriateness* of the emotion and of its expression"[21].

In our daily life, when we are interacting with somebody and realise that our state of mind is not helping us, we could ask ourselves: "Considering that I am about to get angry, how much could I be conditioned by this type of reaction?" Or we could ask: "I'm getting angry, and therefore the people that can see me now could alter their own emotions as well, predisposing them to anger: what could the effect of this be?"

By focusing on these simple questions, we have actually significantly modified our reaction: some time has gone by (a few seconds), which has contributed to defusing it and we have brought to the fore a type of rationality that takes into account the effect that we would have on others. We could call it a *functional* self-control, directed towards what we wish to achieve.

If we go further, we could consider how both enthusiasm and a co-operative attitude are other attributes increasingly in demand. These are "competencies" that every company director would like to find among his or her employees, but that are not so easy to find. Why is that? Once again it probably has something to do with faulty strategies. When you observe somebody, how can

21 Quoted by Daniel Goleman, *Emotional Intelligence: Why It Can Matter More Than IQ*, Bantam Books, 1996.

you tell if he or she is enthusiastic about what they are doing? The answer is that you simply deduct it from their manner and attitude. And it is a perfectly valid answer! Indeed enthusiasm is something that is immediately noticeable, as it is equally *contagious*. Given the naturalness of these processes, we could be fooled into thinking that everything is extremely easy, but in reality we could write a whole book on how to enthuse and motivate people. However, we are in danger of getting off the subject: what matters to us in this context is that others do notice our enthusiasm and that consequently it must be equally straightforward to detect any potential 'lack of enthusiasm' on our part, with all its implications. We do not even need to ask ourselves what the preferred choice should be: would you really like to employ in your firm someone who is not enthusiastic?

We would now like to draw this chapter to a close with a final reflection on an aspect that we have always regarded as fundamental for a team or a group that shares a common purpose, namely co-operation. We could define it as the tendency of an individual to work in a team by providing his positive contribution to a common objective. We could therefore deduct that co-operation is an absolutely crucial trait for a leader, a manager and an executive; once again, it is absolutely paramount to take the mirror effect into account. Just try to imagine a manager at a very important meeting for which he has been preparing really hard, someone with years of experience and highly skilled, who a few minutes before the meeting discovered that his wife may have betrayed him. Do you think that, irrespective of his outstanding abilities, this manager will be able to hide his emotions from the people in front of him? The incongruence, which in this case would be huge, between his desire to conclude the meeting successfully and his inner state, in a hurry to sort things out with his spouse, will be only too noticeable given the way he talks, the way he moves and looks at his watch, the way he breathes: all messages that reach mirror neurons without being filtered and which will have a specific impact on the people at the receiving end of these observations. More than one of them will surely notice that: "The boss was a bit odd today...", or will comment, "Did you noticed something wrong with him today?" These are messages that we constantly pick up, with extraordinary speed and effectiveness.

The war of the neurons

What is interesting is that, having this automatic imitation mechanism, we often predispose ourselves to unwittingly copy the negative emotions and behaviour that we encounter on a daily basis. Everybody knows how difficult it is to work in a place where the human environment is very negative. One of the most stressful things about work is dealing with colleagues who are negative, who bring their personal problems to work and do not hesitate to talk about them, thereby infecting their fellow workers. Do you know anyone like this?

Companies invest large sums of money in their staff training, often teaching advanced communication skills, problem solving and motivational training techniques. But all that is required is for one single individual who has not taken in these teachings to show up at work one morning at 8 a.m. sporting his or her *usual face* to trigger off a dangerous "rogue wave" capable of potentially plunging the whole firm into sadness.

The fact is that every day we face a rather strange

'arm wrestling' challenge between neurons. This is how it works: each time we encounter someone whose emotions are very different from ours, we unleash a challenge between neurons. Eventually one of the two will end up winning, the one whose emotions are more congruent than the other, or more deeply rooted, including in a negative sense too.

If, for instance, we encounter someone whose outlook is very pessimistic, who focuses on the negative side of everything and constantly conjures up negative scenarios, we will be facing quite a difficult challenge: which one of us is going to infect the other?

When we face someone whose conviction of his or her own emotional state is deeply ingrained, the only weapon at our disposal is to generate (beforehand) a positive frame of mind and be convinced of it (but not artificially!), while waiting for the other person to be directed by us. When he or she gives in (and they will, sooner or later...) they will be the ones imitating our way of being and they will probably say things like: "Hey, how do you always manage to be so positive?" because they will not like our being so calm. It is at this point that the 'arm wrestling' comes in: do not let go of your state now but keep it up, because it could well result in a: "Know what? Talking to you is really nice! I really needed that." You will have won the arm wrestling competition.

Continue to enjoy your positive frame of mind, while waiting for the 'contagion' to set in fully, because if you relax your guard now, the other's negativity can instantly force you back into his or her 'field' with a simple: "You can afford to be positive because you're not as desperate as me". At this juncture the word 'desperate' alone could draw you towards despair. Words possess indeed an enormous power: simply saying: "we have a problem" makes us worry, without waiting to see if a problem actually exists. Likewise, in the face of our colleague's alleged 'despair', we risk immediately falling into the trap. It will therefore come down to our willpower and to our frame of mind to ensure that we are the winners of this little battle.

If, in responding to the last sentence of this negative person, we were to say something along the lines of: "Gosh, with so much despair, how much chocolate do we need to eat to feel better?" we would make a 'nice diversion' from their attempt to bring us down and the situation would remain firmly within our control. Our influence would continue to exert a hold on this negative person (who is extremely well trained, so you need to train well too!)

It certainly looks easy, but being equipped with a prompt answer that would instantly bring about a 'positive zone' is a difficult and demanding task, which requires constant training. However, one thing is sure: it is definitely worth it!

CONCLUSION

Our intention was to demonstrate the extent to which the discovery of mirror neurons and the Mirror System can radically modify both our daily lives and the way we view interpersonal communication. This *empathic* and *practical* thread that unites us with everyone else–which constantly involves us in communicative relationships, whether we like it or not–brings us extraordinarily close to each other and destroys the illusion that we can remain *isolated*. When we are with others, we *are* them, in that we share the meaning of both our actions and our emotions.

We live in a society that is busy asking questions that often distract from that most profound sense that ties individuals to their existence. Co-operation and the spread of feelings of love and generosity appear increasingly more distant and remote from mass feelings, and the media is busy administering massive daily dose of negative and violent messages, full of extremely poor social values.

The kind of knowledge that pertains to mirror neurons, to this *wonderful mechanism of ours*, makes clear to us that a type of social responsibility is present in each moment of our lives, as each individual person or group of people puts a part of themselves into society: each person interfacing with someone else can become "infected" with their emotions. We are all active players within this system and we add our emotions to it; the system subsequently decides whether to imitate all or part of these emotions of ours or to do away with them altogether.

Therefore, we need to think about the opportunities that this discovery presents to each of us, within the context of society, the workplace, or the family. Let us think for a moment about the business environment: the time has come to regard company personnel as an investment. Have you ever walked into a shop only to come across shop assistants whose off-hand attitude reveals that they are patently 'tired' of working in an environment that perhaps does not appreciate them, does not adequately reward them financially and does not satisfy them? This is something that we come across very often and it is certainly not a strongpoint of a commercial enterprise. Are employers aware that if they began to appreciate their employees they could ensure that they did their jobs with a smile on their faces? And if the employees were smiling (and we are talking about a sincere smile!) the number of clients would definitely increase, resulting in an immediate increase in profits.

The sales staff and the reception clerk, together with the cashier and the entire front office staff, are the best advert for any business that deals with the public and as well as offering products and services, they also offer the opportunity to reach a state of mind. Customers visiting the shop can not only examine the merchandise on display or discuss the services on offer: they are also exposed to the influence of the employees' emotional state. We often choose a particular bank instead of another on the grounds of the *quality* of its cashiers; and what we mean by quality is what is *inside* them, because it is noticeable! The same applies to supermarket staff, waiters, bartenders and telephone operators, because mirror neurons are activated by sounds and the use of words too. How many clients would a supermarket lose, despite a regular influx of thousands of people, if they suddenly decided to put a demotivated individual on the checkout? We could also calculate how many clients they could gain by investing in training courses aimed at boosting their employees' morale, arising from the awareness that they are emotion 'spreaders'.

Try to imagine a newly recruited employee, a young man whose CV is impeccable but who is quite grumpy and causes arguments amongst the staff by fuelling interpersonal issues. Was recruiting him such a good idea? What is his true cost to the company? The time will come when, more than the actual CV, what will be truly crucial is the emotional state that the new recruit contributes to the corporate environment, and at that point companies will be genuinely willing to invest in the corporate 'climate', given that this is the real heart of the workplace, together with good ideas and proper management. We are talking about aspects that are different from mere 'know how': what will matter more and more in the labour market will be those attributes that are linked to the 'know how to be', such as self-control, the proper management of one's emotional states, the ability to understand others' emotions, and the ability to co-operate. These are all potential skills that are not easy to impart, in that they are independently developed by following a personal evolutionary path. The job market will be increasingly discerning when it comes to the distinction between 'know how' versus 'know how to be'; to us this looks like a positive step, especially these days when science is providing us with very accurate answers on how interpersonal relationships tend to evolve. Perfect organisational and management strategies, promoted by high-calibre managers, are totally powerless against the spread of frustration or sadness. It is the emotional state that prevails over any communication technique: even the best speakers or salepersons are not very effective if their inner emotional state is abysmal because, as we have seen, it is clearly noticeable.

This is true especially when it comes to the family environment, where we are all involved in creating the highest possible level of peace, given our collective awareness of how critical this is. The emotional framework that is established through interaction between family members makes a decisive contribution towards the creation of a good family 'climate'. The mother who *shouts*: "Calm down!" at the child will not be rewarded with calm, rather with *more shouting, or with the fear of shouting.* Eating together sitting around the dining table only to observe a family member who is either sad or frustrated will generate a negative feeling in everyone who is present, which will undoubtedly reduce the precious pleasures of domestic conviviality.

Or let us consider education: knowing that each child *experiences naturally within himself or herself* the same emotional framework as the adults with whom he comes into contact immediately places a tremendous amount of responsibility on each of the adults, namely the responsibility of leaving a significant emotional mark in the child's life. What emotions do we wish to etch into the heart of the children with whom we have established a connection?

Similarly, being aware that the child, through observing adults, recognises, or learns to recognise, *what they are doing,* means we should pay a great deal of attention to each movement that we make in front of children.

It is thus of paramount importance that, before we carry out any action, we are fully aware of the emotional framework that we are inevitably communicating at that precise moment, just as it is equally crucial that we fully realise what we are getting across to others *by doing whatever we are doing*. This represents just a small effort that can lead to great results, especially because we are now perfectly aware that others know what we are doing and they experience what we are going through. The recognition of the emotional state that we carry inside ourselves, knowing that it is visible and that it can potentially be imitated, enables us to find our bearings in the best possible way when it comes to interpersonal relationships. It is simple: anyone who looks at us and therefore experiences negative emotions obviously does not want anything to do with us. On the other hand, having implemented an effective strategy to re-establish a positive frame of mind, we could experience the fantastic feeling of noticing positive changes in those we meet, simply because they have observed us. These same people will be attracted by our emotional state, meaning that they will be infected by it: the more positive, peaceful, balanced and *congruent* it is, the more people will feel inclined to want to be in our company.

ABOUT THE AUTHORS

Matteo Rizzato is a professional coach, certified in NLP New Code. His passion for the discovery of mirror neurons has made him an experienced researcher of excellence in relational dynamics. He is a consultant to companies, schools, sports and top managers. For more information: matteorizzato.wordpress.com.

Davide Donelli is a medical student at the University of Parma. His painstaking research and his wish to make the mirror neuron mechanism as widely accessible as possible led him to Professor Giacomo Rizzolatti and Matteo Rizzato. The fruit of these meetings is the book that you are holding in your hands.

ACKNOWLEDGEMENTS

We would like to offer our heartfelt thanks to Professor Giacomo Rizzolatti for both his precious advice and patience, and for his great generosity, as well as our warmest thanks to Catia Fantini for the splendid illustrations that accompanied the first Italian edition of this book.

We would also like to thank all those who have given us so much throughout this fascinating journey, especially John, Pietro, Rudi and Regina, Andrea, Daniele, Eletta, Verilde and Alessandro.

BIBLIOGRAPHY

Donato M., *I bambini ci educano,* Armando Editore, Roma 2010.

Ekman P., Friesen W.V., *Unmasking the Face. A Guide to Recognizing Emotions from Facial Expressions,* Malor Books, 2003.

Ekman P., *Emotions Revealed: Recognizing Faces and Feelings to Improve Communication and Emotional Life,* Holt & Co., 2004.

Gazzaniga M., Ivry R.B., Mangun G.R., *Cognitive Neuroscience: The Biology of the Mind,* 3rd Edition, W.W. Norton & Co., 2008.

Goleman D., *Emotional Intelligence: Why It Can Matter More Than IQ,* Bantam Books, 1996.

Gray's Anatomy: The Anatomical Basis of Clinical Practice, Churchill Livingstone, 2008.

Iacoboni M., *Mirroring People: The Science of Empathy and How We Connect with Others,* Picador, 2009.

Morris D., *Manwatching: A Field Guide to Human Behavior,* Harry N. Abrams Inc., 1979.

Rizzolatti G., Sinigaglia C., *Mirrors in the Brain: How Our Minds Share Actions, Emotions, and Experience,* Oxford University Press, 2008.

Rizzolatti G., Vozza L., *Nella mente degli altri,* Zanichelli, Bologna 2008.

Russell T., Senior C., Gazzaniga M.S., *Methods in Mind*, The Mit Press, 2006.

Watzlawick P., Weakland J.H., Fisch R., *Change: Principles of Problem Formation and Problem Resolution*, W.W. Norton & Co., 1974.

Young B., Lowe J.S., Stevens A., Heath J.W., *Wheater's Functional Histology: A Text and Colour Atlas*, 5th Edition, Elsevier, 2006.

MORE…

Have you enjoyed this book?

An interview with the Author about this book with English translation is available here:

- www.blossomingbooks.com/en/books/i-am-your-mirror.php

And, of course…

we have more titles in the pipeline!

Watch this space!

www.blossomingbooks.com

HANDS OFF OUR HOLY TERRORS.
Empathic care of children with ADHD (Attention Deficit Hyperactivity Disorder)
Emilia Costa and Daniela Muggia

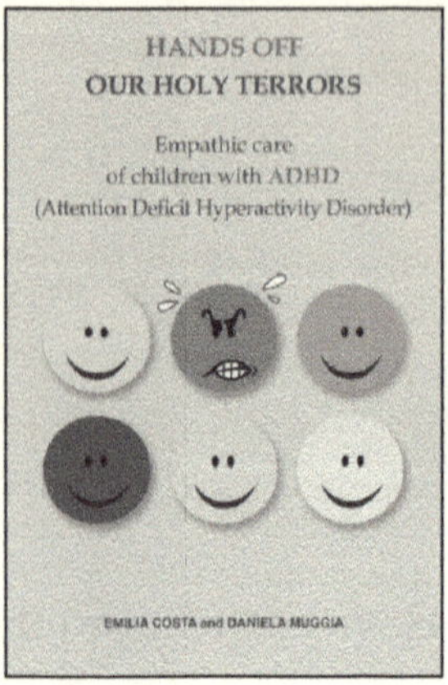

ADHD is Attention Deficit Hyperactivity Disorder, a syndrome whose reality is in doubt today. Children diagnosed with it are often subjected to heavy and risky therapies based on psychopharmacological drugs. **What if there were another, non-invasive, way to help them?**
The innovation of this approach is threefold:

- it takes into account the new paradigm introduced by the evolution of **studies about empathy** (we can have more information if we are in a suitable state to grasp it, and at the same time we can communicate the state of great peace that we can train ourselves to attain);
- it introduces the concept of a collective "**mandala of suffering**" (the child, the parents, the teachers, the therapist or the carer);
- passing through any of these people, it inserts into the well-oiled mechanism of self perpetuated suffering a transformative element that brings this process to a halt.

The inspiration comes from the method ECEL®, Empathic Care at the End of Life, which derives from **the marriage of Tibetan thanatology and neuroscience**. It is based on a state of great empathy that characterizes not only the dying but also children. And that the carer can learn to rediscover in themselves through training. A wealth of resources and scientific information is available in this book.

Professor Emilia Costa*, author of over 360 scientific publications, many of them pioneering, studied directly under Jung, Assagioli and Tedeschi. She teaches psychiatry and psychotherapy at La Sapienza University in Rome and is also Dean of the Scientific Committee of Pharmacovigilance on the over prescription of drugs to children, promoted by "Hands off the Kids", an important Italian association.*

Daniela Muggia, thanatologist*, winner of the 2008 Terzani Award for the Medical Humanities, studied under Sogyal Rinpoche for almost 30 years. After over 20 years of volunteering with the terminally ill, she has developed the method ECEL®, Empathic Care at the End of Life, one of the most popular courses in hospitals, hospices and masters degrees in palliative care in her Country.*

START WITH THE HEART.
A new medical model
Silvia Di Luzio

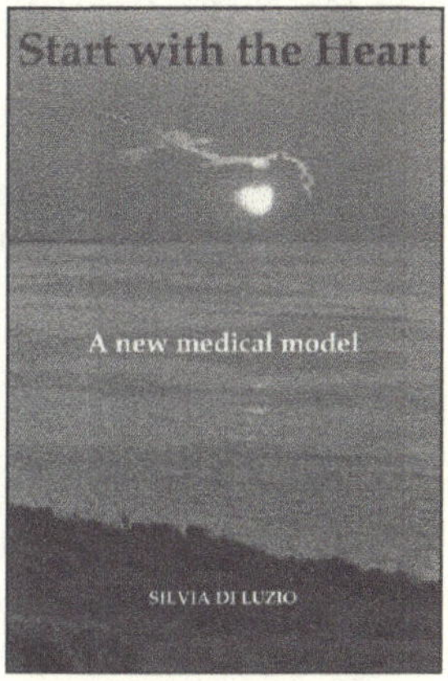

An established cardiologist, sensitive to medicine's current needs, explains how the answer may come literally... from the heart. Today, medicine itself and the concepts of both "health" and "treatment" must be revisited from a different standpoint, where the patient is not simply a machine, but the interconnection between body and spirit. The author presents an extraordinary record of various case histories through which she has personally verified this interconnection, showing how the physical side has healed by working with the spiritual aspect. As part of the overall picture, the heart is not just an effective and powerful symbol of a well-organized society, but it also represents the meeting point for both body and emotions, due to physiological reasons. This therefore makes the heart the key towards reaching a new concept of total healing. The book is accompanied by a supporting review of the latest news and publications related to this new healing concept; a field in which the author has trained very thoroughly.

***Silvia Di Luzio** is a cardiologist and Senior Research Associate at the University of Chicago, USA. Having worked in hospitals, nursing homes and sports-related associations, she combines her medical experience with her longstanding training with Anthony Robbins. She has also trained in both PNL and psycho-oncology at Prof. O. Carl Simonton's school.*

2012-2021 THE DAWN OF THE SIXTH SUN.
The Path of Quetzalcoatl
Sergio Magaña (Ocelocoyotl)

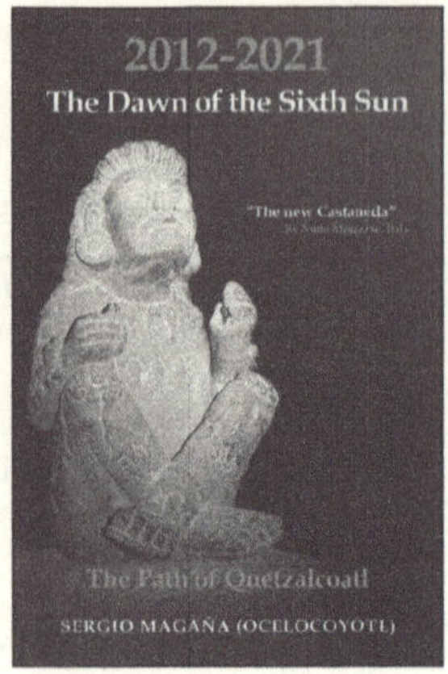

"It is entirely remarkable that pre-Colombian people of Mesoamerica have foreseen the release of the wisdom we need to master this transformation precisely now, when it is actually taking place . . . including concrete practical instructions on how to master our body and our mind to cope with the challenge that awaits us."

–ERVIN LASZLO, Nobel Prize Nominee, author and founder /president of the Club of Budapest.

"...Sergio Magaña has been entrusted with the sacred task of revealing once-secret knowledge on the transformation of the Earth and humanity, both collectively and individually, as the Age of the Sixth Sun unfolds..."

–Daniel Pinchbeck, author of *2012: The Return of Quetzalcoatl*

"This is not a book to read. This is a book to study. Take it seriously!"

–GAY LUCE, Founder of Nine Gates Mystery School

What happens on and after December 21, 2012? There has been much confusion and many predictions based on the Mayan calendar. Some people think time on Earth will end . . . but what if there were an intact, unadulterated, and compete resource from the ancestors that gives us the wisdom we need for the shift, and an understanding of the coming era?
According to Toltec /Aztec tradition and calendar, the movement from the Fifth to the Sixth Sun is a shift in human consciousness—our understanding of how we relate to self, each other, the Earth and the cosmos. The Sixth Sun brings a new energy that represents an opportunity. We have a choice. We can either move toward our further destruction, or along a path to manifest our highest nature. In order to bring back balance and live from a state of grace, there is individual inner work to be done. The breathing exercises, poses, and other ancient practices contained in this book are based on cosmic mathematics and provide access to altered states of consciousness and new ways of being needed for this transition.

Sergio Magaña "Ocelocoyotl" *is a well-known and respected teacher of the 4,000-year-old Toltec tradition of Mesoamerica, including the Tol shamanic lineage of dreaming knowledge (nahualism) passed on from master to student for 1,460 years. He lives in Mexico City.*